PRAISE FOR
STATIN NATION

"In my experience, statin drugs are the number one cause of iatro-
genic (doctor-caused) disease in the United States. For those who
want proof, I suggest they read *Statin Nation*. Justin Smith doesn't
fall for the usual "coronary artery plaque is the only cause of heart
disease" mantra. That theory—and its attendant drugs, stents, and
bypasses—has been a boondoggle for the medical-industrial complex but not so helpful for people. In *Statin Nation*, Smith carefully
and accurately assesses this misguided theory, comes to more well
founded conclusions, and helps his readers find their way to more
productive approaches to preventing and treating heart disease.
Well done."

—THOMAS COWAN, MD, author of *Human Heart, Cosmic Heart*

"This book amalgamates and updates the author's two *Statin Nation*
documentaries, which are also highly recommended. It provides a
succinct but comprehensive discussion of the fallacies of the lipid
hypothesis of coronary heart disease. It explains why neither cholesterol nor saturated fats cause heart attacks and why there is no
such thing as 'good' or 'bad' cholesterol. Abundant references for
those who want additional information."

—PAUL J. ROSCH, MD, clinical professor of
medicine and psychiatry, New York Medical College;
chairman of the board, The American Institute of Stress

"A complete and authoritative explanation of the causes of heart disease. Smith's presentation explains why statin therapy is ineffective and dangerous, and why the cholesterol hypothesis is obsolete and disproven by scientific evidence. This book fills an important need for a comprehensive explanation of the pharmaceutical industry's efforts to profit from statin drugs, of the trivial effect on prevention of heart disease by these drugs, and of their serious toxic side effects. More importantly, the book describes the true causes of heart disease and emphasizes optimal nutrition as the correct approach to prevention."

—KILMER MCCULLY, MD, author of *The Heart Revolution*

"Our utmost wealth is our health. Accordingly, *Statin Nation* demonstrates that lifestyle changes are the cornerstone of good cardiovascular health, and that the supposed benefits of widely used heart medicine—lauded by industry-sponsored research—are based on flawed science. I concur with Justin in this effort to warn our population about the dangers of statin drugs."

—SHERIF SULTAN, PhD, professor of
vascular surgery, National University of Ireland;
president, International Society for Vascular Surgery

$TATIN
NATION

$TATIN NATION

The Ill-Founded **War** on **Cholesterol,**
What Really Causes **Heart Disease,**
and the Truth About the Most
Overprescribed Drugs in the World

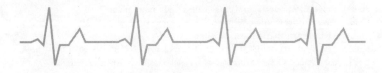

JUSTIN SMITH

Chelsea Green Publishing
White River Junction, Vermont

Project Manager: Patricia Stone
Project Editor: Michael Metivier
Copy Editor: Deborah Heimann
Proofreader: Helen Walden
Indexer: Ruth Satterlee
Designer: Melissa Jacobson

Printed in Canada.
First printing November, 2017.
10 9 8 7 6 5 4 3 2 1   17 18 19 20 21

Our Commitment to Green Publishing
Chelsea Green sees publishing as a tool for cultural change and ecological stewardship. We strive to
align our book manufacturing practices with our editorial mission and to reduce the impact of our
business enterprise in the environment. We print our books and catalogs on chlorine-free recycled
paper, using vegetable-based inks whenever possible. This book may cost slightly more because
it was printed on paper that contains recycled fiber, and we hope you'll agree that it's worth it.
Chelsea Green is a member of the Green Press Initiative (www.greenpressinitiative.org), a nonprofit
coalition of publishers, manufacturers, and authors working to protect the world's endangered
forests and conserve natural resources. *Statin Nation* was printed on paper supplied by Marquis that
contains 100% postconsumer recycled fiber.

Library of Congress Cataloging-in-Publication Data
Names: Smith, Justin, 1971– author.
Title: Statin nation : the ill-founded war on cholesterol, what really causes heart disease, and the
   truth about the most overprescribed drugs in the world / Justin Smith.
Description: White River Junction, Vermont : Chelsea Green Publishing, [2017]
   | Includes bibliographical references and index.
Identifiers: LCCN 2017031861 | ISBN 9781603587532 (paperback) | ISBN 9781603587549 (ebook)
Subjects: LCSH: Statins (Cardiovascular agents)—Popular works. | Hypercholesteremia—
   Physiological aspects. | Heart—Diseases—Prevention. | Heart—Diseases—Alternative treatment.
   | BISAC: HEALTH & FITNESS / Diseases / Heart. | HEALTH & FITNESS / Alternative
   Therapies. | MEDICAL / Pharmacology. | MEDICAL / Drug Guides.
Classification: LCC RM666.S714 S65 2017 | DDC 615.7/18—dc23
LC record available at https://lccn.loc.gov/2017031861

Chelsea Green Publishing
85 North Main Street, Suite 120
White River Junction, VT 05001
(802) 295-6300
www.chelseagreen.com

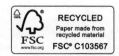

CONTENTS

PREFACE

In 2001, I left my well-paid job as an account manager for a data analysis company in England, and started an intensive diploma in personal fitness training and sports massage therapy. After completing the course, I worked as a personal trainer and massage therapist within the corporate fitness industry and then as a freelance personal trainer at the BBC in London until 2009. During those eight years, I was very fortunate to work with an incredibly diverse range of clients, every one of whom taught me something new. The various challenges of my work also required a considerable amount of continued education. Luckily, I've always been fascinated by nutrition, which became the subject of a large part of my independent research as well as of several formal courses I took over the years.

What I learned—from my independent research, my nutritionist colleagues, and from my clients—was that much of what we are told about healthy eating is wrong. In fact, in some cases, only when the conventional advice is turned on its head does it resemble something close to helpful. One issue in particular that repeatedly came up was cholesterol. Both in discussions with clients and through my own research I found that highly touted low-fat diets do not work for most people, and in 2006 I read Dr. Uffe Ravnskov's classic text *The Cholesterol Myths*.

Further independent research led to a profound feeling of disappointment with the health care industry in general. I had left my corporate career in order to work in a field that I thought would be less governed by commercial interests and politics, only to quickly realize how naive I had been. I was shocked by the discrepancies between what we the general public are told and the actual scientific evidence. It became obvious that what we think about a wide range of health issues is determined by commercial interests and by experts who are more interested in preserving their own careers than properly informing the public.

In 2009, I published my first book challenging the cholesterol hypothesis. However, those with vested interests continued to heavily promote the false idea that cholesterol causes heart disease. In 2010, I decided to make a documentary film, *Statin Nation: The Great Cholesterol Cover-Up*, about the issues surrounding cholesterol, which was released at the end of 2012 and was well received. This enabled me to make *Statin Nation II: What Really Causes Heart Disease*. During that time I also completed the Guardian Masterclass in investigative journalism. Both films together include interviews with eighteen of the world's leading experts on the issues surrounding cholesterol and statin medications—experts from the United Kingdom, the United States, Denmark, Sweden, France, Lithuania, Australia, Egypt, and Japan.

While some information is best presented on screen, other information can only be presented in a book. The information contained in this book is based on nine years of research, in-depth interviews completed during the making of the *Statin Nation* documentaries, and correspondence with a number of other scientists and researchers.

Introduction

Worldwide, heart disease is the leading cause of death, and for decades, health authorities have promoted the idea that it is caused by dietary fat and cholesterol "clogging up the arteries." As a result, cholesterol-lowering medications—the class of drugs called statins in particular—have become, by far, the most widely used intervention for the prevention of heart attacks. As of this writing, an estimated thirty-five to forty million people in the United States, seven to eight million people in England, and millions more people worldwide now take statins.[1]

Doctors make prescribing decisions about statins based both on cholesterol guidelines set by health authorities and on the results of various cardiovascular disease risk calculators. The latest guidelines and risk calculators suggest that at least one billion of the world's adults are eligible for statins. The guidelines and risk calculators derive from a model of heart disease that considers such risk factors as age, cholesterol levels, high blood pressure, obesity, gender, family history, ethnicity, smoking, and diabetes.

This book will argue that the risk factor–based model of heart disease and the associated risk calculator currently in use are both deeply flawed, designed to serve the interests of the pharmaceutical industry rather than the health of patients. In fact, the current approach serves to unnecessarily convert millions of healthy people into patients. Some of the risk factors are valid, but some are not, and the focus on a short list of suggested risk factors neglects the underlying, genuine causes of heart disease. However, before decon-structing the current approach it is worth making a few background remarks about evidence-based medicine, which to some extent gave rise to the risk factor–based approach.

Medical doctors once relied on their intuition, experience, and familiarity with individual patients, in addition to medical knowledge, when making clinical decisions. However, there was not a great deal of documented evidence to support many of the interventions that they used. During the 1990s the concept of evidence-based medicine was adopted, and since then it has been rapidly implemented in most industrialized countries. Evidence-based medicine involves the inte-gration of scientific evidence from the medical literature into clinical practice. Most people agree that evidence-based medicine is a good thing, and it is considered a significant step of progress within med-icine, but few people are willing to talk about its negative aspects.

One problem with evidence-based medicine is that the evidence is based on populations of people rather than on individuals. The results of a clinical trial might show that a group of people who were given a particular medication had fewer heart attacks. There-fore, the evidence suggests that the medication should be considered for everyone who has similar physical and medical characteristics as those people who were included in the clinical trial. Unfortunately, this approach overlooks the fact that not everyone can be expected to benefit from the medication. In the clinical trial, some people would have benefitted, some would have experienced no benefit, and others might have been harmed, even though on average there was an overall benefit. For example, clinical trials of statin medica-tions have shown that about 1.6 percent of people benefit. Which means of course, that 98 people or fewer out of every 100 who take the medication do not receive any benefit, and are instead only being exposed to potential adverse effects.[2]

An individual person has no way of knowing which category they will fall into: the 1 percent who will benefit, or the 99 percent who will not benefit. And if a patient does experience adverse effects from the statin, these adverse effects could be considered an acceptable trade-off because the clinical trials create the impression that the patient *will* benefit.

This is one aspect of what authors Erik Rifkin and Edward Bouwer refer to as "the illusion of certainty" in their book of the same name.[3] In essence, the illusion of certainty refers to how the human brain interprets numbers, risks, and probabilities. A positive result from a clinical trial, to most people, means that the drug being tested has been found to "work." It is easy to ignore or forget the fact that it only worked for a percentage of people, and very often only a tiny percentage of people.

During the last few decades both doctors and the general public have increasingly sought published data to support interventions, marking a huge step in the right direction. We tend to view the data as reliable, authoritative, and final, which in some cases it is. However, there is a great deal of scope for misunderstandings, misuse, and even abuse during the interpretation of the data. Drug companies, for example, fund most clinical trials, which means that these companies own the data, which in turn means that the data can be presented in ways that suit commercial objectives rather than the interests of the patient.

Coinciding with the implementation of evidence-based medicine has been the expansion of clinical guidelines. In theory, this makes sense. If the data provides evidence that a treatment works, then why not set clinical guidelines based on this evidence in order to make clinical practice more efficient and help more patients? The problem is that if the data has been skewed to serve commercial interests, all the guidelines do is effectively scale up the misrepresentation of the data. In addition, the setting of clinical guidelines provides an opportunity to focus the attention of doctors and patients into specific areas at the neglect of other areas; for example, doctors might become so focused on driving down cholesterol that they do not have sufficient time to talk to their patients about physical activity, stress reduction, or other important lifestyle changes.

To make things worse, in some countries doctors' performance in general practice is now measured in terms of the impact it achieves at the population level rather than on individual patients—for example, by calculating the percentage of a doctor's patients who are within the recommended limits for blood pressure and cholesterol levels. This approach can work relatively well if the intervention in question has been shown to benefit most people. However, not only statins but also a number of other medications currently in use have been approved based on only a tiny benefit at the population level.

Experts who support the mass prescription of statin medications suggest that a small reduction in heart attack risk, if applied across a large population, is quite significant. Applied nationwide, a 1.6 percent reduction in risk equates to the prevention of thousands of heart attacks. But the other side of the argument is that for every one hundred people given the medication, twenty could suffer significant side effects.[4]

When setting clinical guidelines, health authorities tend to look at the upside and downplay the downside. In addition, the experts who set the guidelines often have connections with drugs companies. Where cholesterol-lowering guidelines are concerned, at least half of the experts on the panel setting the guidelines have direct financial links with the pharmaceutical companies that make cholesterol-lowering statins.[4-6] Perhaps we should not be surprised, then, that the threshold for what is considered an ideal cholesterol level has always been lowered with each update to the guidelines, making

millions more people eligible overnight for statins and other cholesterol-lowering medications that are in the pipeline.

In theory, doctors still have the flexibility to make clinical decisions
for individual patients, but in practice, guidelines are implemented
based on the best (supposedly) clinical evidence, so doctors feel
obliged to follow them. Not following the guidelines could be seen
as not implementing "best practice," and in some cases this can lead
to disciplinary procedures. The guidelines are also used in some
countries, such as the United Kingdom, to set performance-related
pay schemes for doctors, creating a financial incentive that is inter-
twined with the guidelines.

The risk factor–based model of heart disease lends itself to the setting of clinical guidelines. It involves establishing numerical targets
or thresholds for each of the identified or suggested risk factors. The
cardiovascular risk calculator used by the American Heart Association
takes into account gender, age, total cholesterol and HDL cholesterol, blood pressure, ethnicity, smoking, and diabetes status.[7] The
relevant data for each of these "risks" is entered into the calculator;
the generated result is supposed to accurately reflect the probability
of the individual having a cardiovascular problem within the next ten
years. In general, if the result is a 7.5 percent or higher chance, the
person is deemed eligible for a cholesterol-lowering statin.

That this calculation overestimates risk has been widely
reported.[8] The calculator captures more people into the statin eligibility category than it should, due to an error in its formula. For
while smoking, being male, advanced in age, and having diabetes all
increase the risk of cardiovascular disease, cholesterol is not a valid
risk factor.[4,5,9–16] High blood pressure is part of the body's response
to the problem, not the problem itself.

In 2011, a study was published in the *Journal of the American
Medical Association* that should have led to a complete reappraisal

of the current risk factor–based approach, but instead it was largely ignored. The study included more than 500,000 people who were admitted to the hospital with a first heart attack but without any prior cardiovascular disease.[17] The researchers looked at five of the traditional risk factors in relation to survival after this first heart attack: high blood pressure, smoking, high cholesterol, diabetes, and family history of heart disease. This list of risk factors is similar to those in the aforementioned risk calculator used by the American Heart Association.

If such risk factors were reliable as predictors of mortality, then we would expect that people with more of them would have worse rates of survival. However, the reverse is true. In this study, the more risk factors a person had, the more likely they were to survive their first heart attack. In fact, greatest risk of death was associated with having *no* risk factors; people with none of the five risk factors were 1.5 times more likely to die after a heart attack than people who had all five.

How can someone with no risk factors have a worse outcome than someone who smokes and has high cholesterol, high blood pressure, diabetes, and a family history of heart disease? It is only possible if the current risk factor–based approach is flawed or is missing other important factors that contribute to heart disease but are not included in the current model. This book will show that this is indeed the case.

Many of the real causes of heart disease have been known for a long time but have been clouded over by the eagerness of health authorities to medicate healthy people. In addition, some specific nutritional interventions have been shown to be at least six times more effective than statin medications. And studies have shown that stress reduction could be as much as eleven times more effective than statins. Yet very few people know that these more effective and much safer alternatives exist.

I hope that after reading this book the reader will have a better understanding of the flaws in the current model of heart disease, the true nature of the condition, and the alternatives to statin medications. Armed with this information, readers should be empowered to have more detailed discussions with their doctors and to make informed decisions about their own health.

This book does not claim to have included all of the factors and complex interactions that contribute to heart disease. It is unlikely that all of the real causes have been identified, since the false assumptions made by health authorities have led to decades of misdirected research. However, I hope that sufficient information is included here to present a completely different way of thinking about heart disease that goes well beyond the misguided war on cholesterol.

CHAPTER ONE

The Etiology of Heart Disease

*For every complicated problem there is a solution
that is simple, direct, understandable, and wrong.*

H. L. MENCKEN

Problems associated with the heart and blood vessels are responsible
for 30 percent of all deaths worldwide. Of the multitude of heart
conditions that can affect us, most are said to be the result of coronary heart disease (CHD), also sometimes referred to as coronary
artery disease (CAD), which affects the larger blood vessels that supply blood and oxygen to the heart muscle (see figure 1.1). In people
suffering from CHD, the walls of these arteries become thickened,
narrowing the space available for the flow of blood and oxygen.

For decades, the public was presented with a model of heart disease that suggested dietary fat and cholesterol somehow get stuck
to the inside walls of the arteries, forming a fatty plaque and accompanied by the formation of blood clots. As the disease progresses, a
blood clot can eventually completely block an artery, obstructing the
flow of blood and oxygen to the heart, resulting in a heart attack.

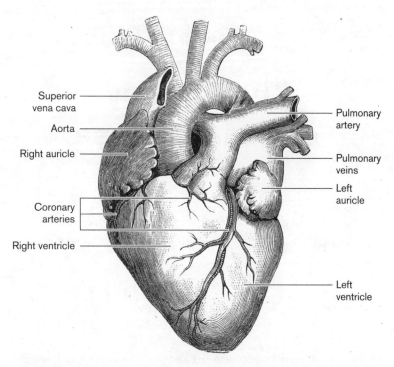

Superior vena cava

Aorta

Right auricle

Coronary arteries

Right ventricle

Pulmonary artery

Pulmonary veins

Left auricle

Left ventricle

Figure 1.1. Basic anatomy of the heart and coronary arteries.

Over time, more people became aware that CHD actually involves a thickening of the arterial wall, and not fat and cholesterol simply getting stuck to the inside wall of the artery; so our current basic model has slightly evolved. Health authorities now acknowledge that the process associated with developing CHD involves initial damage to the lining of the artery wall. However, health authorities still believe that fat and cholesterol are two of the main causes of this process. The British Heart Foundation, for example, states: "Too much bad cholesterol in your blood can cause fatty material to build up in your artery walls."[1] The idea that dietary saturated fat increases blood cholesterol levels, eventually causing heart attacks, is known as the diet-heart hypothesis, a hypothesis that has never actually been proven.

The scientific process, of course, involves the generation of hypotheses that are then tested in order to determine if they are valid. Almost every time the diet-heart hypothesis has been tested, it has been found to be false. This might come as a surprise to many readers, considering the ubiquitous message from health authorities that we must avoid dietary saturated fat, as well as the billions of dollars that are spent each year on cholesterol-lowering medications. However, as we shall see, the diet-heart hypothesis is perpetuated not for the purpose of improving peoples' health, but for the purpose of generating profit for the pharmaceutical and food industries.

The Diet-Heart Hypothesis: A Short History

At the beginning of the twentieth century, Nikolai Anitschkow, the Russian pathologist, conducted experiments that involved feeding rabbits huge amounts of cholesterol purified from egg yolks dissolved in plant oils.[2,3] The rabbits developed extremely high blood cholesterol levels and arterial plaques. These findings have often been quoted as supporting the diet-heart hypothesis; however, because rabbits are vegetarian, they do not normally consume foods containing cholesterol, and therefore they do not possess the relevant metabolic machinery to metabolize cholesterol and excrete excess cholesterol through the liver. In addition, a few years after Anitschkow's experiments, I. B. Friedland found that high cholesterol levels could be avoided by giving rabbits thyroid hormone along with the high quantities of cholesterol.[4]

The diet-heart hypothesis only started to gain prominence after Ancel Keys, a well-known and highly influential physiologist based at the University of Minnesota who advised the US Department of Defense during World War II, published research in the 1950s and 1960s. Keys formulated meals for combat soldiers that became known as K-rations, but he is equally known for his now infamous study of six nations published in 1953.

In that study, Keys plotted the dietary fat intake of six countries against the numbers of deaths from heart disease in those countries on a graph.[5] The graph showed a straight-line relationship between higher fat intake and increased heart disease mortality. However, at the time of the study, data points were available for sixteen other countries, which Keys omitted from his graph. Had they been included, the direct relationship would have completely disappeared and no meaningful connection would have been seen between dietary fat and heart disease.[6] Despite this obvious flaw, the study is still quoted today in support of the diet-heart hypothesis.

Over time, glaring contradictions to the diet-heart hypothesis began to emerge, most notably in the early 1990s in what became known as the French paradox. Researchers noticed that people living in France consume much more saturated fat than people in England and the United States, yet their rate of heart disease is drastically lower. Obviously, this was inconvenient for supporters of the diet-heart hypothesis, so it was decided that the French are protected from their hazardous diet by their consumption of red wine. Some epidemiological data does support the notion that drinking red wine can offer some protection against heart disease; however, drinking alcoholic beverages of any kind moderately is associated with a lower risk of heart disease. There is nothing uniquely protective about red wine. Moderate drinkers are also likely to take a moderate approach to other aspects of their life, such as exercise, stress, and the amount of food they eat. A moderate, rather than excessive, lifestyle is likely to produce a range of health benefits.

France is not the only paradox. People in Iceland also consume more saturated fat than people in England, but die from heart disease at about half the rate. In Denmark, people eat less saturated fat than people in Iceland, but the Danes have a higher rate of heart disease deaths. Similarly, the Portuguese consume about one third less saturated fat in their diet than the French, but have a higher rate of heart disease deaths. People in Lithuania consume half as much saturated fat as people in England but Lithuania has almost double the rate of heart disease deaths. In fact, looking at global data in the same way that Ancel Keys did, we find many more countries that contradict the diet-heart hypothesis than support it.

Health authorities state that saturated fat should make up less than 7 percent of our total caloric intake. Yet very few countries have such a low saturated fat intake. Lithuania does, and it has one of the highest heart disease death rates in the world.[7]

Despite the flaws of the diet-heart hypothesis, we have been made to fear cholesterol to the extent that it has now become synonymous with heart attacks, concurrent with the perception that societal cholesterol levels have increased as a result of poor lifestyle choices. However, cholesterol levels were declining in most developed countries since 1960, before the war on cholesterol was initiated. Cholesterol-lowering statin medications didn't start to become more widely used until the mid-1990s. Between 1960 and 1994, average cholesterol levels in the United States decreased by about 18 mg/dL (0.46 mmol/L). Other countries, such as Finland and New Zealand, also experienced similar reductions in cholesterol.[8] This might not seem like a significant amount; however, between 1999 and 2006 in the United States average cholesterol levels only reduced 4 mg/dL (0.11 mmol/L) despite twenty-eight million people taking a cholesterol-lowering statin at that time. So, if cholesterol levels were already declining at a greater rate than has been achieved by statins,

why are tens of millions of people told that they need statins? Before
we answer that, let's take a closer look at cholesterol.

The "Good" and "Bad" Cholesterol Fallacy

Most people are familiar with the concept of "good" and "bad" cholesterol. High density lipoproteins (HDLs) are considered "good"
and low density lipoproteins (LDLs), such as those warned against
by the British Heart Foundation, are "bad." These designations are
quite remarkable considering the fact that HDLs and LDLs are not
really cholesterol.

Cholesterol does not mix with water; therefore, in order for it to
be transported through the bloodstream it has to be carried inside
something called a lipoprotein. A lipoprotein is an assemblage of
fats, protein, and other substances that move around the body.
Lipoproteins carry a number of very important materials that are
needed by the body's cells, and they also participate in the immune
system. HDLs and LDLs do contain cholesterol, but they also contain CoQ10, vitamin E, beta-carotene, and other substances. The
cholesterol found in HDLs is exactly the same as the cholesterol
found in LDLs. The explanation we are given for HDLs being
"good" and LDLs being "bad" is related to their direction of travel
within the body.

Most cholesterol is made in the liver. LDLs transport cholesterol
from the liver to the cells, including those cells in the walls of coronary arteries. HDLs transport cholesterol back to the liver. It might
seem logical to suggest that LDLs are bad because they transport
cholesterol to artery walls. However, this is a normal and vitally
important function of the body. All cells need cholesterol, which is
a major component of the cellular membrane. Cholesterol makes
cells waterproof; cells need to be waterproof in order for the internal

structure of the cell to be protected from its external environment. Therefore, a mechanism is required to enable all cells to get the cholesterol they need. LDLs provide this important mechanism.

Cholesterol is an interesting molecule. It is often called a fat, but chemically speaking it should be called an alcohol, though it does not behave like one.[6] The complex structure of cholesterol provides the protection cells need. When cells become damaged, they require cholesterol to help repair the damage. A discussion of the tissue repair qualities of cholesterol can be found in scientific literature at least as far back as 1975.[9,10] However, this important issue is conveniently ignored by those who support the idea of good and bad cholesterol.

There are a large number of reasons why cells within the walls of the arteries that supply blood and oxygen to the heart might become damaged. Smoking cigarettes, high blood glucose levels, stress, and toxicity, for example, can all cause this type of damage to the arteries. In response to this the body might need to make more cholesterol, which it sends to the cells that need it via LDLs. LDLs might even be required in greater numbers in order to perform this function more efficiently. But this is the effect of the problem and not the cause. Suggesting that LDLs cause heart disease is like blaming traffic police at the scene of a motor vehicle accident. Yes, the police are there, but to clear up the incident, not because they caused it.

In addition, questions remain about the suggested link between higher levels of LDLs and heart disease. We are told that, mathematically, people with higher LDL levels have a greater risk of heart disease, but this, in fact, is not true. Supporters of the cholesterol hypothesis point to cholesterol-lowering clinical trials where a significant decrease in LDL levels occurred at the same time as a slight reduction in the risk for heart problems. However, LDL reduction is not necessarily the reason for the slight reduction in heart problems. There are many other biochemicals that are affected by cholesterol-lowering statins. For example, it is widely known that statins have an anti-inflammatory effect, and that they could help improve iron metabolism and potentially help stabilize plaques within arteries. The slight reduction of heart problems could be due to a wide range of potential effects that have nothing to do with LDL levels. I am not suggesting that cholesterol-lowering statins are good; we shall see later in this book that the overall risk-benefit profile of statins is not favorable for most people. My intention here is simply to make the point that medications have a wide range of effects and it can be difficult to determine exactly which effect produces a specific result.

A large study published in the *American Heart Journal* in 2009 found that the level of so-called bad cholesterol is actually lower in people with heart disease, not higher. The study included around 137,000 people from 541 hospitals in the United States who had been admitted to the hospital with heart disease, all of whom had their LDL level measured within twenty-four hours of admission.[11] The researchers found that the average LDL level for this group (104 mg/dL (2.7 mmol/L) was actually lower than the average level for the American general population (123 mg/dL [3.3 mmol/L]).[10,12,13] In addition, people admitted to the hospital after a heart attack with lower levels of LDLs also have a higher risk of dying within the first thirty days[14] and also in the next three years.[15] And, in general, people live longer with higher cholesterol levels.[16–19]

All of this data raises an obvious question: If people with heart disease have lower levels of so-called bad cholesterol, why are some countries around the world spending billions of dollars each year lowering these levels?

Some cardiologists admit this major flaw in the current model, but not always on the record. During the filming and research for my documentary film *Statin Nation II*, I visited countries with both low and high rates of heart disease in order to gather some clues about the real causes of heart disease, including Greece, or more specifically, the island of Crete.

Crete is one of many examples of places in the world where people consume large amounts of fat and cholesterol yet have a very low rate of heart disease. By chance, I sat next to a cardiologist on the flight to the island from Athens. When I told the cardiologist of my interest in including Crete as a case study in the documentary, he responded "We are told that LDL particles cause heart disease, but no one has ever proved it."

As this anecdote suggests, increasing numbers of people are now aware that fat and cholesterol are not the culprit.[16-24] Some, however, have simply replaced the diet-heart hypothesis for the inflammation hypothesis, which is a step in the right direction but one that still does not provide an adequate explanation for the real causes of heart disease.

Heart Disease and Inflammation

Arterial plaque contains a range of substances. Fat and cholesterol are present, but so are monocytes and macrophages (white blood cells associated with inflammation), and cytokines (small proteins that have specific effects on cell-to-cell interaction), T lymphocytes (T-cells, white blood cells that increase in the presence of an infection), and other substances.

It is now widely accepted that the overall process associated with the buildup of arterial plaque is inflammatory. Any injury to the inside wall of an artery leads to a blood clot and the inflammatory response. Heart disease could therefore be thought of as *coronary arteritis*; although this might not describe the complete process, it is more meaningful than the simple "artery clogging" description still being perpetuated.

Endothelial cells that make up the lining of the arteries contain sensors that read how hard the blood pushes and pulls as it rushes through the blood vessels; the arteries can, in a sense, "feel" the blood flowing through them. These endothelial cells also have the ability to adapt to specific changes in the local environment, regulate artery wall remodeling, and regulate the release of immune factors. Generally, endothelial cells keep everything balanced and under control in the blood vessels and arteries.

Endothelial cells also coordinate the recruitment of inflammatory cells to the site of injury or infection. This understanding of the way that endothelial cells coordinate the inflammatory response, and the presence of other key substances related to inflammation, has led to the somewhat erroneous belief that heart disease is caused by inflammation. It is important to keep in mind that the inflammation is the local reaction to injury, and the real causes of heart disease are those factors that actually cause the injury itself or hinder the body's ability to deal with the injury and return the artery wall back to a healthy state.

As mentioned earlier, damage to the artery wall causes blood clots to form along with the development of arterial plaque. If the process continues and the body is not able to restore the condition of the artery back to a healthy state, a blood clot can eventually completely block an artery, causing an occlusion (closing of the artery). The heart tissue downstream of the occlusion is then deprived of blood and oxygen and the heart muscle cells in that area die, causing an area of necrosis, or a heart attack.

Blood clots are certainly a common feature of heart disease and heart attacks. In *Statin Nation II* it was suggested that the process associated with heart disease could more accurately be described as arterial *clotting* rather than arterial *clogging*, and people on both sides of the statins debate agree that blood clotting is a central, key aspect of the disease. In fact, arterial plaques have even been described as blood clots in various stages of repair.[25]

The processes involved in blood clotting as a result of arterial damage are complex; the best explanation can be found in the chapter "Cardiovascular Disease Is Primarily Due to Blood Clotting," written by Dr. Malcolm Kendrick as part of the excellent book, *Fat and Cholesterol Don't Cause Heart Attacks*, edited by Professor Paul J. Rosch.

However, the purpose of this chapter is to raise an important question regarding the order in which the events take place: Are blood clots in an artery the cause of a heart attack or the result? This might seem strange to ask but there is reason to think that blood clots can form in the arteries as a result of damage to the heart muscle itself. And data exists to support this hypothesis.

The conventional model suggested by experts who support the cholesterol hypothesis is presented largely as a simple plumbing problem: Over time, the pipes that supply the heart with blood and oxygen become blocked by fat and cholesterol. And interventions are mostly aimed at keeping the pipes clear. However, there are a number of other features of heart attacks that must be considered:

- The plumbing approach does not consider the many factors that can affect the condition of the heart muscle itself. As we shall see, the strength and health of the heart muscle itself is affected by a large number of lifestyle and nutritional factors in addition to the condition of the arteries.
- Psychological and physical stress changes physiology in a profound way that not only leads to the accumulation of arterial plaque but also directly damages the heart itself.

- The electrical control system of the heart that provides the impetus for the pumping action is also affected by stress, with nutritional status and certain environmental factors also having an effect.
- It has been demonstrated that the heart brings into prominence the collateral circulation in response to, and hence compensating for, a blocked artery.

Some researchers have suggested that, in the case of severe heart attacks, blood clots form as a secondary feature, after the heart attack rather than before it. Therefore, we are left with a classic chicken-and-egg scenario. What comes first, the heart attack or the blood clot(s)? This is discussed in a little more detail in the following section.

Giorgio Baroldi

Giorgio Baroldi was an Italian cardiovascular pathologist who for half a century challenged the conventional theory regarding the processes associated with heart disease. Baroldi wrote a large number of research articles, and his work was published in some of the most respected medical journals in the world. However, as has happened in many other instances within medicine, his challenges to conventional wisdom fell upon deaf ears.

In 2004, Baroldi, along with coauthor Professor Malcolm Silver from the University of Toronto, published a book that contains a detailed summary of an alternative view of how heart disease develops.[26] One of the key issues discussed by Baroldi is that in the presence of a blocked artery the heart adapts by increasing blood flow through the collateral circulation. Most people are familiar with the basic anatomy of the heart shown in figure 1.1. This kind of image is widely used. However, what we usually do not see in this representation is the collateral circulation. The collateral circulation consists of an intricate network of blood vessels that also supply the heart muscle with blood and oxygen.

Baroldi made a number of observations that led him to conclude that a blocked artery might not be the most important factor in a heart attack, or at least that the occlusion is not the only factor. Baroldi observed that:

1. Some people have a significant amount of narrowing of the artery without any signs of damage to the heart muscle itself. And the narrowing could have existed for years without any clinical symptoms of heart disease.
2. There is no relationship between the extent of coronary artery disease and the degree of damage to the heart muscle itself. Logically, we would expect that if there were a greater extent of arterial plaque or occlusion, then the area of dead heart muscle tissue would also be greater. However, Baroldi concluded that the extent of arterial disease did not correlate with the degree of actual damage to the heart.
3. It is possible to have an infarct (an area of dead heart muscle tissue) without a corresponding occlusion.

Other researchers have also come to similar conclusions. Dr. Knut Sroka, a general practitioner in Hamburg, Germany, has assembled a website containing detailed research on the mechanisms associated with heart disease.[27] Dr. Sroka suggests that "complete acute blockage of a coronary artery is found in only about 50% of heart attacks."[28]

If blocked arteries can be circumvented by the collateral circulation, and there is not a connection between the extent of artery disease and the size of the area of dead heart muscle tissue, then heart attacks could start from within the heart itself rather than as a result of arterial damage. This hypothesis is sometimes referred to as the myogenic theory of myocardial infarction. A pioneer in this field was Dr. Quintiliano H. de Mesquita,[29] a Brazilian physician and scientist, whose work has been continued by fellow Brazilian Carlos Monteiro, an independent researcher and scientist.[30]

The myogenic theory raises questions about common surgical procedures that are currently being performed, such as coronary bypass surgery and the insertion of stents. These interventions are based on the idea that a blocked artery will always lead to a heart attack. If that is not the case, then some people might be having costly unnecessary surgical procedures.

In simplified form, the myogenic theory of heart attacks starts with psychological and physical stress causing an imbalance in the nervous system. This imbalance in turn changes the quantities of various biochemicals that are released, and the heart muscle becomes overly reliant on the burning of sugar for energy instead of fat, creating an acidic environment that affects the contractility of the heart muscle. This dysfunction can lead to a localized area of cell death (necrosis)—a heart attack.

Once the heart attack has occurred, the fluid dynamics of the arteries change, which can cause the inside walls of the arteries to become damaged. The body responds to this damage to the arteries by forming a blood clot, and the arteries are then subject to the same processes associated with the buildup of arterial plaque. If arterial plaque does build up, the resultant narrowing of an artery can make the situation worse by further impeding the supply of blood and oxygen to the heart muscle. The condition will eventually present as arterial plaque, possibly a full occlusion, disruption to the electrical control system of the heart, and an area of dead heart muscle tissue. But what was the main culprit, and which one came first?

There are still a considerable number of unknowns regarding the precise mechanisms involved in the development of heart attacks, and in what order they appear for each individual person. However, acknowledging these unknowns does not prevent us from understanding the real causes of heart disease or from knowing what to do in order to aid recovery after a heart attack.

As we shall see, the best approach for preventing a heart attack, or recovering from one, is to look at the factors that affect all areas of heart function: the condition of the arterial wall, the health of the heart muscle itself, and the electrical control mechanism of the heart. And, in fact, what we find is that the most important real causes of heart disease do indeed affect all of these areas. But before we get to these causes of heart disease, it is worth looking at the benefits of cholesterol, as well as revisiting the question of why, if higher LDL levels are associated with a lower risk of heart disease, do we spend so much energy and money on cholesterol-lowering medications like statins?

CHAPTER TWO

The Importance of Cholesterol

As mentioned in chapter 1, a great deal of effort has been directed toward educating the general public about the "dangers" associated with cholesterol. It is fair to say that the supporters of the diet-heart hypothesis have been very successful in creating a fear of cholesterol-as-artery-clogger, a fear greater even than that of heart disease itself. Despite this fearmongering, evidence suggests that high cholesterol levels can be extremely beneficial.

We have known for some time that high cholesterol in elderly people is associated with longer life. This was the conclusion of a study completed by a team of researchers at Yale University School of Medicine.[1] Researchers in the Netherlands also found that life expectancy increases when cholesterol levels are higher; those with higher cholesterol levels appear to be better protected from both cancer and infection.[2]

A number of studies have found high cholesterol to be protective for elderly people with heart failure.[3-8] An article published in *The Lancet* concluded that lowering cholesterol levels is detrimental in patients with heart failure.[9]

Further evidence that higher cholesterol protects against infections was established by Professor David Jacobs and Dr. Carlos Iribarren, who tracked the health of more than 100,000 healthy individuals in the San Francisco area for fifteen years: Those who had low cholesterol at the start of the study had a higher rate of infectious disease.[10] Another study published in *The Lancet* looked at cholesterol levels and death rates in more than 3,500 elderly Japanese-American men over a twenty-year period. The study confirmed what had been found in previous studies: an increase in death rates in people with low blood cholesterol levels. The authors went on to say that not only do these results provide more evidence that low cholesterol in the elderly is associated with an increased risk of death, but also that people who maintain low cholesterol over a twenty-year period have the worst outlook for mortality.[11]

Higher levels of cholesterol could also protect against Parkinson's disease. A study published in the journal *Movement Disorders* found that people with Parkinson's disease had lower LDL levels than people who did not have the disease.[12]

A study published in the *Journal of the American Medical Association* analyzed data from 122,458 patients enrolled in fourteen international clinical trials.[13] The authors compared the frequency of various risk factors in people who had heart disease. They found that only 39 percent of all men and 34 percent of all women who had heart disease had high cholesterol or high triglycerides. If cholesterol was assessed independently of triglycerides, this percentage might have been even less, suggesting that low cholesterol is seen more often than high cholesterol in patients with heart disease.

Researchers at Boston University investigated the relationship between total cholesterol levels and cognitive performance in 789 men and 1,105 women.[14] They discovered that low cholesterol levels were associated with lower performance in tests for word fluency, concentration, and overall cognitive performance.

We are constantly learning more about the important functions in which cholesterol plays a role. Research led by the University of California, for example, has confirmed that derivatives of cholesterol play an important role in the immune system and could protect humans from a wide range of viruses, such as Ebola, Rift Valley fever, Nipah, and other deadly pathogens.[15]

When the immune system is first exposed to a new pathogen, it develops the ability to recognize the invader when it next enters the body by producing memory cells. This "memory" of the immune system is provided by a clustering of T-cell receptors. A study published in *Immunity* and *Journal of Biological Chemistry* found that cholesterol plays a key role in this process.[16]

Cholesterol provides the raw material for making vitamin D, all of the steroidal hormones, and bile acids for digestion. And, as already stated, a large proportion of our cellular membranes are made up of cholesterol. Cholesterol (along with saturated fat) provides the structural rigidity that cells need in order to work properly. And we also now know that cholesterol plays an important role in cellular signaling, or the "intelligence" of the cell.[17]

Cholesterol is important for all cells but particularly for cells associated with the brain, the nervous system, and the immune system. Scientists at the Karolinska Institute in Stockholm, Sweden, and Swansea University's College of Medicine in the United Kingdom have identified two steroid-type molecules, cholic acid (a bile acid) and 24S,25-Epoxycholesterol (a derivative of cholesterol), that play an important role in the survival and production of nerve cells in the brain.[18]

Dietary Studies and
the Diet-Heart Hypothesis

A fundamental aspect of the diet-heart hypothesis is that dietary saturated fat increases blood cholesterol levels, and more specifically, LDL levels. As we've seen, the correlation between LDL levels and heart disease has yet to be proven, as there are instances where low levels of LDLs are associated with a greater risk. However, leaving that part of the discussion aside, it is worth looking specifically at the suggested link between dietary saturated fat and LDL levels.

A study published in the The Lancet involving 1,420 people analyzed data collected during the U.K. National Diet and Nutrition Survey.[19] The researchers found no connection between saturated fat and the level of LDLs. They also found no connection between saturated fat and total cholesterol levels.

A study published in the New England Journal of Medicine[20] compared the effects of a low-fat diet with a high-fat diet. The study's participants were split into two groups, one for each diet. The people in the high-fat-diet group were asked to follow the Atkins Diet,[21] which advocates consuming large amounts of saturated fat from animal proteins. After one year, each group was assessed for risk factors associated with heart disease. There was no significant difference in total cholesterol levels or LDL levels between the two groups. In addition, the group following the high-fat Atkins Diet showed a significant increase in HDL (good cholesterol) levels.

In 2008, a similar study was published in the New England Journal of Medicine. In this two-year study three different diets were compared: a low-carbohydrate/Atkins-type diet (high in fat content), a Mediterranean-type diet (with moderate fat content), and a low-fat diet. Again, the researchers found no link between increasing the amount of saturated fat in the diet and LDL levels.[22]

Another study compared a low-fat diet with a high-fat diet in women who were overweight but otherwise healthy.[23] At the end of the six-month study, there were no significant differences in cholesterol levels between the two groups. The people in the high-fat-diet group had eaten twice as much saturated fat, yet their total cholesterol was unchanged, their LDL levels were unaffected, and their "good cholesterol" (HDLs) had increased slightly. The authors of the study even stated: "This study provides a surprising challenge to prevailing dietary practice."

In yet another study comparing a low-carbohydrate diet with a low-fat diet,[24] the people in the low-carbohydrate-diet group were instructed not to eat more than 30g of carbohydrate per day (just slightly more than is allowed on the Atkins Diet). The majority of the food eaten in the low-carbohydrate-diet group would have contained significant amounts of saturated fat. At the end of the one-year follow-up, changes in both total cholesterol and LDL levels were not significantly different between the groups. And "good cholesterol" (HDLs) had decreased more in people who followed the low-fat diet.

Finally, in another study comparing low-fat and high-fat diets,[25] the people in the low-fat-diet group were instructed to eat a diet containing no more than 10 percent saturated fat. The people in the high-fat-diet group were allowed to eat as much saturated fat as they liked, and unlimited eggs. The level of LDLs did not differ statistically when the results were analyzed. The most significant difference between the two groups was that the high-fat diet increased HDLs. Similar results were seen in yet another study published in the *Journal of the American Medical Association*, which compared four weight-loss diets representing a spectrum of low-fat to high-fat diets.[26]

Other studies have looked at not just cholesterol levels but actual incidences of heart disease, in the context of different amounts of saturated fat. For example, a study published in the *American Journal of Clinical Nutrition* included 75,521 women who were followed for ten years in order to determine the effects of different diets.[27] The primary aim of the study was to determine the effect of increasing the glycemic load of the diet, which relates to the impact each diet has on blood glucose levels, but the amount of saturated fat was also recorded. The women in the group that ate the least amount of saturated fat had 186 cases of heart disease whereas those with the highest amount of saturated fat intake had 139 cases.

Researchers from Harvard University investigated the effects of different diets on the progression of heart disease in 235 women who already had heart disease. The women were followed for around three years. As in the studies mentioned earlier, the researchers found that saturated fat intake was not related to LDL levels. They also found that greater saturated fat intake was associated with less progression of heart disease, whereas poly-unsaturated fat and carbohydrate intakes were associated with a progression of heart disease.[28]

There have also been several large studies in the form of meta-analyses that have combined data from multiple studies. These studies have also failed to find a connection between saturated fat intake and cardiovascular disease.[29–32]

Cholesterol and the Thyroid

Although cholesterol levels in the general population of America have on average been declining, there are, of course, some cases where an individual person's cholesterol level has genuinely increased. It is important to keep in mind that cholesterol levels can and do fluctuate significantly in healthy people, and cholesterol levels can be different depending on the time of year (they tend to be higher in the winter months). But when an individual person's cholesterol level has increased significantly over time, the first thing that should be considered is the function of the thyroid gland.

The thyroid, positioned near the front of the neck, is a butterfly-shaped gland responsible for metabolism, body temperature, growth, and brain development. The thyroid gland secretes various hormones; the main one is thyroxine (known as T4). We have known for at least eighty years that blood cholesterol levels increase when there is a deficiency of thyroid hormone. According to Dr. Broda Barnes, a pioneer in the diagnosis and treatment of thyroid disorders,[33] the connection between cholesterol levels and a deficiency in thyroid hormone was so close in the 1930s that it was suggested that blood cholesterol levels could be used as a diagnostic test for thyroid function.

Low thyroid levels increase cholesterol levels and also increase the risk for a range of heart problems. However, both heart problems and increased cholesterol levels are caused by a sluggish metabolic rate, as well as a range of other effects due to low thyroid function. In fact, both high and low thyroid levels can cause heart problems.[34]

In 1877, Dr. William M. Ord conducted an autopsy examination of a women whose thyroid gland was replaced by connective tissue. Ord found that the entire arterial system showed atherosclerosis. The arteries supplying her kidneys, brain, and heart all contained a buildup of plaque. He also found a swelling of the skin and the connective tissues, which—unusually—did not release water at the cut surface, as is found in cases of fluid retention due to kidney failure. Ord suggested that the absence of the thyroid gland was the cause of these conditions. The tissues with the high water content contained an unusual amount of mucin, a thick, glue-like substance. Ord coined the term *myxedema* to describe these water-logged tissues. During the next decade, other physicians reported a number of similar cases of myxedema where the thyroid gland had been removed.[33]

At the turn of the twentieth century, various experiments were performed on sheep and goats that involved removing their thyroid glands, after which they developed plaques in their coronary arteries. However, animals that had their thyroid removed but were also given thyroid hormone did not develop arterial plaques. Heart attacks had not yet been described clinically, so these important findings were almost forgotten.

In recent years, however, medical literature has again acknowledged the connection between low thyroid function and high cholesterol,[35,36] but there is not much evidence that doctors are exploring this as a cause of high cholesterol before starting a statin. Thyroid problems are common in many countries, and so this issue should certainly be given more attention.

CHAPTER THREE

The Business of Selling Drugs

If cholesterol doesn't cause heart disease, it is logical to question why so many people, including so many doctors, believe that it does. This question can be answered through an appreciation of the general environment in which doctors now work, of which almost every aspect is controlled by drug companies. Most of us know this intuitively, but it is useful to break down and examine the main areas of this commercial influence. There are a number of significant problems with medical journals and the way medical research is published. Few people have the time or the inclination to investigate these problems; however, these issues directly affect all of us and distort our perception of the safety and effectiveness of medications such as statins.

Pharmaceutical companies are a business just like any other, and the people who work for these companies naturally want to increase profitability. Shareholders also want to see a return on their investment. These companies, of course, want to sell more drugs every year, and they have been very successful in doing so.

For example, the Office for National Statistics in the United Kingdom publishes data concerning the number of prescriptions written in England. The years between 2005 and 2015 saw a 50 percent increase in the number of prescriptions, and during 2014 to 2015 there were more than one billion prescriptions.[1] In the United States, around $330 billion is spent on pharmaceuticals each year. Some might argue this is simply an indication that new drugs are being made available to patients. In some cases that might be true; however, overall, the increase in the number of prescriptions is due to marketing efforts by drug companies and not the appearance of genuinely beneficial drugs.

In his book *The Trouble with Medical Journals2*,[2] published by The Royal Society of Medicine, Richard Smith analyses the problems and current trends in medical publishing, based on his experience working for the *British Medical Journal* (BMJ) for twenty-five years, and serving as editor and chief executive of the BMJ Publishing Group from 1991 to 2004, when he became, arguably, one of the most influential people in medicine. Smith's book provides a fascinating and highly readable account of medical research–related issues, and is recommended to anyone who wishes to gain an insight into the world of medical research and how it influences our daily lives. Smith does not specifically examine the subject of cholesterol, but he does explain how the pharmaceutical companies have been experiencing a productivity crisis. In order for these companies to grow and increase profits, they need to develop innovative drugs that genuinely provide significant benefits for patients. Unfortunately, such pharmacological breakthroughs have been much fewer than was hoped for.[2]

The number of new drugs approved in the United States by the Food and Drug Administration (FDA) had diminished,[2] and pharmaceutical companies were forced to look for other ways to achieve business growth, including increasing marketing efforts to get more people to take existing drugs, and creating new diseases by lowering the threshold for the definition of high blood pressure and high cho-lesterol: basically, converting healthy people into patients.

Some authors describe such activities as disease mongering, the "invisible and unregulated attempts to change public perceptions about health and illness in order to widen markets for new drugs."[3,4] In an article published in the *Public Library of Science (PLoS) Medicine*,[4] Dr. Barbara Mintzes, an Australian research scientist who specializes in the study of pharmaceutical policy, describes the various forms that disease mongering by pharmaceutical companies can take. They include:

- Promotion of anxiety about future ill-health in healthy people
- Exaggerating the number of people affected by a disease
- Promotion of aggressive drug treatment for mild symptoms
- Introducing new conditions that are hard to distinguish from normal life, such as social anxiety disorder
- Promoting drugs as the first solution for problems previously not considered medical, such as disruptive classroom behavior or problematic sexual relationships

Disease mongering exploits our deepest fears of suffering and death, and lucrative professional careers have been built on this exploitation and the pursuit of new diseases.[5] Increasingly, emphasis is placed on suggested risk factors for a disease rather than on the disease itself. High cholesterol has become synonymous with heart disease and some studies have focused solely on cholesterol levels, including a study in England that looked at how many people have low HDL levels compared with how many people are taking cholesterol-lowering drugs,[6] as well as one examining HDL levels in various European countries.[7] Since low HDL levels are thought to contribute to the risk of developing heart disease, investigations such as these might seem valid. However, collectively, they create the impression that having the suggested risk factor is the same as having the disease itself, especially when researchers use this type of data to conclude that more people need to take statins or additional drugs that specifically target HDLs, a conclusion reached with no consideration of the many real factors that contribute to heart disease. By looking solely at one of the suggested risk factors, we lose sight of the main objective, and studies conducted on raising HDL levels with medications have thus far in each case resulted in an increase in deaths.

Doctors and Drug Companies

In recent years, drug companies have been restructuring their organizations, shifting more of their resources into marketing and "education." In research-based drug companies, for example, the number of people employed in research and development has fallen while those in marketing have increased.[2] Almost all of the major drug companies now spend more on marketing activities than on research to find new treatments.

The majority of the expenditures on sales and marketing are directed not at consumers but at health professionals. About $24 billion is spent each year on marketing drug products to health care professionals, and it has been estimated that 99 percent of doctors use information provided by pharmaceutical companies in their clinical practice.[5] If the number of prescriptions (and therefore profits) were not affected by this sales activity, pharmaceutical companies would not do it.

Of course, pharmaceutical companies should be allowed to sell their products to doctors, as a necessary part of the health care process. However, connections between doctors and drug companies can become inappropriate and have an unnatural influence on prescription habits. This is particularly true when doctors in influential positions, who determine treatment protocols, are supported by pharmaceutical companies. Prior to 2004, for example, a cholesterol level above 250 mg/dL (6.5 mmol/L) was considered high, but in 2004 the guidelines were changed and the definition of high cholesterol became 200 mg/dL (5.0 mmol/L), making millions more people eligible for statins overnight. Eight out of the nine experts who decided on the new definition of high cholesterol had connections with drug companies that make statins.[8]

The cholesterol guidelines were again changed in 2013; it was decided that people should be given a statin based on their overall risk rather than their cholesterol level. But the threshold for the overall risk was lowered. Previously, if someone had an estimated 20 percent or higher overall risk for a cardiovascular problem within the next ten years, then they were considered eligible for statins, but in 2013 the threshold was lowered to a 7.5 percent overall risk. A new risk calculator was also implemented, which raised considerable controversy because it quickly became obvious that the new risk calculator was suggesting statins for millions of people who clearly did not need them. Many doctors refused to use the new calculator. Half of the panel members who decided on the new risk calculator, including the chairman and one of two co-chairs, had connections with statin manufacturers.

According to a survey completed in the United States, 94 percent of doctors have some kind of link with the pharmaceutical industry.[9] The frequency of different types of connections was found to be:

- 83 percent receive food and drinks from a pharmaceutical company in the workplace.

- 78 percent receive drug samples from a pharmaceutical company sales representative.
- 35 percent are reimbursed by a pharmaceutical company for costs associated with professional meetings.

Other payments are given for consulting, speaking engagements, service on an advisory board, and enrolling patients into clinical trials.[9,10] Some doctors say that these ties with industry do not influence the prescribing of drugs; however, it is generally accepted that a social obligation is inherently associated with a gift. People often feel the need to reciprocate when they receive one, even if the gift was unwanted or unasked for.

Likewise, if a doctor receives excellent hospitality from a pharmaceutical company during a seminar or conference, she or he is less likely to be openly critical of the company's products. Doctors are only human. Interestingly, a survey of medical students found that 86 percent thought it was improper for a politician to receive a gift, but only 46 percent thought it was improper for themselves to receive a gift of a similar value from a pharmaceutical company.[11] Links between doctors and drug companies, in theory, could be beneficial; however, most studies have found negative outcomes, such as doctors not being able to identify inaccurate claims made by drug companies; doctors requesting new, more expensive drugs that have no demonstrable benefit over existing ones; increased prescription rates; and irrational prescribing behavior.[10]

Bias in Publishing Results

Clinical trials for drugs are almost always conducted by the pharmaceutical companies themselves. Various studies have found, perhaps unsurprisingly, that when a pharmaceutical company sponsors research into its own drug, the results are considerably more likely to show the drug in a favorable light.[12] In addition, clinical trials that show favorable results are more likely to be published,[13] and pharmaceutical companies have attempted to prevent studies that show unfavorable results from being published.[11]

Take, for example, the ENHANCE trial, which was a two-year trial to test the effects of using a drug called *ezetimibe* in conjunction with a statin to achieve greater reductions in cholesterol. Trial participants were split into two groups; one group was given both ezetimibe and the statin, and the other was given only the statin. LDL levels were reduced to a considerably lower level in the group given both ezetimibe and the statin.[14] According to the cholesterol hypothesis, these greater reductions in LDL levels should have resulted in a greater reduction in the buildup of arterial plaque. However, the researchers found the opposite to be true. Rather than providing any additional benefit, the addition of ezetimibe actually led to a slight increase in the amount of plaque in the main arteries that supply blood and oxygen to the brain.[15]

The results of the ENHANCE trial raise more questions about the idea that cholesterol levels are related to the buildup of plaque in arteries. But this is overshadowed by the fact that the drug companies behind the trial attempted to hide these results from the public for as long as possible. The ENHANCE trial ended in April 2006, but the companies that make ezetimibe, Merck and Schering-Plough, did not report the results until January 2008. Even then, the results were only released after the companies received pressure from the United States Congress[14] and after articles questioning the delay began to appear in the news media.[14,16]

The companies blamed the delay on the complexity of the data. A spokesman for Schering-Plough said the delay was unrelated to the negative findings and that the results were not known until two weeks before they were released. However, deadlines for reporting the results were repeatedly missed, while in the meantime millions of people continued to take the drug unaware of the negative results of the trial.[14] Global sales of the drug were US$5 billion in 2007.[17] In England alone, more than two million prescriptions were written in the two years prior to the release of the results, costing the National Health Service £74 million[17] and an unquantifiable amount of medical harm.

If all of this wasn't bad enough, there were also problems with the registration of the ENHANCE trial. Clinical trials are officially registered in order to prevent researchers from changing the objective of the trial once it is under way, since changes could be made in order to cover up unfavorable results. Notably, the ENHANCE trial was not registered until eighteen months after the trial had ended, and an article in the *Guardian* reported that the objective of the trial was altered in the register.[18]

Subsequent studies of ezetimibe show that the use of this drug in conjunction with a statin increases the risk for cancer.[19] Investigators dismissed this as a chance finding,[20] but significant questions remain.[21] Patients are still expected to continue to take this drug, used under the trade names *Zetia*, *Vytorin*, *Ezetrol*, and *Inegy*, on faith that it is effective, potentially exposing themselves to serious side effects.

The ENHANCE trial is also just one instance demonstrating the problems that can arise when focus is placed on suggested risk factors rather than on the disease itself. In order for heart disease medications to be approved by the US FDA, for example, it is not necessary to show benefits in terms of a reduction in heart disease risk, it is merely necessary to demonstrate that the drug lowers "bad" cholesterol (LDLs).[22] This is a dangerous and risky approach for patients, and it distracts researchers away from finding the true causes of the disease. In the ENHANCE trial the suggested risk factor (in this case cholesterol) was significantly further reduced, but the reduction resulted in no additional benefit for patients. Delaying the results of a trial, or never publishing the results, introduces publication bias. An article published in the *New England Journal of Medicine* that investigated the extent of publication bias in antidepressant drug trials found that 31 percent of the trials had not been published and that almost all of the unpublished trials showed negative results associated with the drug being tested. According to the published studies, 94 percent of trials found favorable results for the drug, but when the unpublished trials were included in the data, only 51 percent of the trials had favorable results.[23]

In February 2008, Professor Irving Kirsch and colleagues conducted a detailed analysis of all the clinical trial data on antidepressant drugs submitted to the US FDA,[24,25] including both published and unpublished data. The conclusion reached was that antidepressant drugs were no more effective than a placebo. This example shows how the effectiveness of drugs can be exaggerated if data about them is not published.

The Media

Since many people do not see their doctor regularly, and consultation times are often short in duration, the media represents the most significant source of health information for a large segment of the population. Medical stories are not easy to report. They must be both accurate and authoritative; journalists need to understand the terminology, physiology, epidemiology, study design, and statistical analysis to keep health news in context for the viewer, listener, or reader.[25] Unfortunately, there are few journalists who meet this standard. In almost all cases the reporting of clinical trial results involves journalists simply copying the press release issued by the pharmaceutical company doing the trial.

In 2012, the British Heart Foundation published a report detailing a wide range of heart disease statistics.[26] One of the highlights was the decline in heart disease deaths seen between 2002 and 2010 in the United Kingdom. Reporting on this, the *Daily Mail* wrote "Wonder drug statins have helped slash heart attack deaths by half, research says"; the *Express* wrote "Proof statins save millions from heart attacks"; and the *Telegraph* wrote "Deaths from heart attacks half as treatment pays off." Anyone reading the British press would be left with no doubt that statins are wonderful. However, the report from the British Heart Foundation that these news articles were based on did not mention statins at all, and statins made no measurable contribution to the decline in heart disease deaths. One can only assume that the British media were spun into believing that statins had played a part in the reduction in heart disease deaths by some careful wording in the press release associated with the publication of the report. Though the heart disease death rate has been declining in the United Kingdom since the 1970s, this is due to fewer people smoking cigarettes and better hospital treatments.

Even worse than this lazy journalism was the unwillingness of these media organizations to correct the error. I contacted each of the newspapers about their respective articles. The *Telegraph* did not reply at all. Giles Sheldrick, who wrote the article for the *Express*, replied: "I can assure you I spoke to several medical experts before the article was published." While the *Daily Mail* acknowledged that they made a mistake, they removed the article from their website with no correction or explanation to its 9 million readers. This is just one of many ways that the public is given false information about the benefits of statins and other drugs. Journalists can easily become mouthpieces for those with vested interests.

Medical Journals:
Powerful, but Problematic

Medical journals have a reputation among the general public as being dull and obscure; however, their content influences the lives of millions. Medical journals not only affect all of the clinical decisions doctors make with individual patients but they also directly influence public health policy. There are a number of serious problems with medical journals related to how they are influenced by pharmaceutical companies.

Pharmaceutical companies influence medical journals in a number of ways, the most obvious of which is through advertising. A large percentage of doctors receive journals such as the *British Medical Journal*, the *New England Journal of Medicine*, and the *Journal of the American Medical Association* for free because of the financial support the journals get from pharmaceutical company advertising. Publishers of medical journals are constantly worried that these companies will cut back on advertising, and they argue that advertising produces a better financial return for the pharmaceutical industry than employing more sales representatives would.[2]

Authorship is another problem. As Elizabeth Wager said, there are four types of lie: lies, damned lies, statistics, and the authorship lists of scientific papers.[27] The list of authors that appears at the top of a medical research paper might not reflect true authorship. Scientific communities call this ghost authorship. Ghost authors are people who have contributed to a research study or been involved in writing the paper but whose names do not appear on the list of authors. There are a number of implications associated with ghost authorship. One of the main concerns is that the ghost author is employed by a pharmaceutical company, representing an undeclared conflict of interest. In one study, 75 percent of trials included were

found to have had ghost authors.[28] In this case the ghost authors
were statisticians employed by the pharmaceutical companies supporting the trials. This is important because clinical trials are often
complex and generate large datasets; the statistical report is a fundamental part of the research and it has a crucial influence on what
is written in the publication summarizing the study. Not declaring
the statistician, and thus hiding their affiliation, deceives the reader
about the role of the supporting company.

Problems also exist with the peer review process of published
papers. Richard Smith explains these problems in detail in *The Trouble with Medical Journals*: "Peer review is at the heart of all science. It
is the method by which grants are allocated, papers published, aca-
demics promoted and Nobel prizes won. Yet it is hard to define . . .
and its defects are easier to identify than its attributes."[2]

Peer review could loosely be described as getting a third party to
verify the accuracy of a scientific paper or to help make a decision
about whether to publish it. Ideally the third party should not be
connected with the research and should have no competing interests, but still should be in a position to technically appraise the
methodology and findings. Richard Smith explains that peer review
sometimes seems to be a simple case of someone saying "the paper
looks all right to me,"[2] and examples of a comprehensive, detailed
review of a paper are difficult to find. These issues of conflicts of
interest and lack of critical review directly impact the quality of
what gets published and can mean that important information is not
published if it is contrary to the belief system of the peer reviewer.

CHAPTER FOUR

The Trouble with Statins

We are told that statins provide huge benefits for the prevention of heart attacks, that they have very few side effects, and that everyone should take them. In reality, the benefits have been exaggerated, the significant side effects have been downplayed, and there are very few people for whom statins are appropriate. This chapter first provides a summary of the clinical trial data before discussing the harms that statins have been shown to cause.

Clinical Trials

Although statins do lower cholesterol, we've now seen how lowering cholesterol is not always beneficial for the body. Measures of effectiveness of statins should therefore be based on heart attack risk reduction and improvement in life expectancy rather than effects on cholesterol levels. Unfortunately, some health authorities have at times been hypnotized by the cholesterol-lowering effect of statins, ignoring the fact that many clinical trials have shown an absence of any net benefit to their use. The benefits of statins are also routinely exaggerated, with the drug being portrayed as a wonder drug or "the pill of life."[1] As we will see, the summary information in clinical trial reports is sometimes written to imply much more overall benefit than was actually achieved.

The AFCAPS/TexCAPS Trial

The AFCAPS/TexCAPS trial included 5,608 men and 997 women with average cholesterol levels and no existing signs of cardiovascular disease.[2] Its aim was to test if a cholesterol-lowering statin was able to reduce the number of first coronary events (for example, a first heart attack). Researchers call this *primary prevention*. This trial is of interest because the people included in the trial were in many ways similar to the average person who is prescribed a statin under the current guidelines.

After five years, the group of people who were given the statin did have fewer heart attacks. In terms of percentages, 3.3 percent of the statin group had a heart attack versus 5.6 percent in the placebo group (a difference of 2.3 percent).

What is of more concern, however, is whether or not the statin drug saved any lives, or rather, extended life expectancy. In the summary of the trial report the authors stated: "There were no clinically relevant differences in safety parameters between treatment groups." Unfortunately, the authors failed to mention the fact that overall, slightly more people died in the statin group (80 people) than in the placebo group (77 people).

The greater number of overall deaths in the statin group can be explained by the fact that there were a greater number of noncardiovascular-related deaths; that is, although the use of the statins significantly reduced LDL "cholesterol," and was associated with fewer cardiovascular-related deaths, more people died from other causes. Sixty-three people in the statin group died from noncardiovascular-related causes, versus 52 in the placebo group. This did not, however, stop the authors from stating that the study confirmed the benefits of reducing LDL "cholesterol."

The ASCOT-LLA Trial

The ASCOT-LLA trial was another primary prevention trial to test the effects of lowering cholesterol with a statin. It included 10,305 people (mostly men) aged forty to seventy-nine years, with high blood pressure or other risk factors for cardiovascular disease, but with average cholesterol levels.[3] As with the AFCAPS/TexCAPS trial, the participants in this trial were typical of those who could be prescribed a statin under current guidelines. The average total cholesterol level of the people included in the study was just under 220 mg/dL (5.5 mmol/L) and the average level of LDL "cholesterol" was 130 mg/dL (3.4 mmol/L).

Researchers often use the term *primary end points* to describe the specific outcomes that will be measured in a trial. The primary end points of the ASCOT-LLA were a heart attack or death due to heart disease. Within the group of people who were given the statin, 1.9 percent had a heart attack or died of heart disease, versus 3 percent of those in the placebo group; the statin reduced the risk by just over 1 percent. Unfortunately, the authors of the report described the results as a 36 percent reduction in primary end points. The authors calculated that the 1.1 percent reduction in risk between the statin and placebo groups was 36 percent of 3 percent. In other words, they used a relative percentage instead of an absolute percentage. This constitutes a manipulation of the data that serves only to make the drug look better. If a person is told that a statin will reduce their risk by 36 percent, they might be inclined to take the drug, but if they are told that in real terms, this 36 percent means a reduction from a 3 percent risk to a 1.9 percent risk, they might think twice about it.

It is interesting to note that although the trial was planned to run for 5 years, the researchers were so happy with these results that they decided to stop the trial after 3.3 years. They believed that they had done enough to prove the benefits of the statin. And if we look at the results for deaths from all causes, we find that there was no statistically significant reduction. Therefore, the statin did not improve life expectancy.

The CTT Trials

In 2005, researchers from the CTT (Cholesterol Treatment Trialists) Collaboration completed an overall analysis of fourteen statin clinical trials, which in total included 90,056 participants with a wide range of different risk factors. Some participants had existing heart disease, other forms of cardiovascular disease, or diabetes, while others had none of these conditions.[4] The aim of the analysis was to investigate the effect of reducing LDL "cholesterol" by 40 mg/dL (1 mmol/L) on various outcomes. It should be noted that 40 mg/dL (1 mmol/L) represents a large reduction in LDL levels, since values are typically low anyway.

The results showed that reducing the level of LDLs by 40 mg/dL (1 mmol/L) reduced the risk of dying from heart disease from 4.4 percent to 3.4 percent. If we look at the data for deaths from all causes, the statin group had an overall death rate of 8.5 percent, compared with 9.7 percent in the placebo group.

The same group of researchers published another study in *The Lancet* in 2008. They used the data from the previous analysis completed in 2005, but this time more specifically looked at the people within the study who had diabetes.[5] Their analysis showed that people with diabetes benefited less than those without diabetes. The statin managed to reduce the number of deaths from all causes in people with diabetes from 11.9 percent in the placebo group to 11.0 percent in the statin group.

The MRC/BHF Heart Protection Study

This study included 20,536 high-risk people who already had heart disease, cardiovascular disease, or diabetes.[6] In this very high-risk group, the use of the statin reduced the heart disease death rate from 6.9 percent to 5.7 percent (a 1.2 percent reduction). In this case, the statin also reduced the rate of deaths from all causes by 1.8 percent (from 14.7 percent in the placebo group to 12.9 percent in the statin group).

The 4S Study

The Scandinavian Simvastatin Survival Study, also known as the 4S study, was completed in 1994. Out of all the trials completed to date, the 4S produced the best results for statin use. Numerous trials have been completed since 1994, costing billions of dollars, but none have produced the same level of results.

The 4S study included 4,444 patients who already had heart disease, many of whom had already had a heart attack. At the end of the trial, 8 percent of patients in the statin group had died versus 12 percent of patients in the placebo group. Put another way, over the course of the six-year study, the patients in the statin group had a 91.3 percent probability of surviving, compared with an 87.6 percent probability of surviving in the placebo group.[7]

The 4S study is often quoted in support of the use of statins, but it is rarely mentioned that no other trial has been able to produce the same results. Also, it is often forgotten that this trial included only extremely high-risk patients. The results in this trial population group cannot be assumed to be the same for the general population where the aim is prevention of a first heart attack (primary prevention). In general, the benefits of statins in primary prevention are lower than in secondary prevention.

The TNT Study

Researchers from the TNT study wanted to determine if increasing the dose of a statin drug would provide more benefit.[8] The study analyzed 5,584 patients who already had heart disease and metabolic syndrome (a condition similar to diabetes). Sixty percent of the people included in this study had already had one heart attack, and more than 80 percent had angina (chest pain due to an inadequate supply of oxygen to the heart muscle). One group of patients was given 10 mg of a statin, and the other group was given 80 mg. After approximately five years, major cardiovascular problems occurred in 13 percent of people in the 10 mg group and 9.5 percent of people in the 80 mg group, a difference of 3.5 percent. Again, the authors chose to describe this as a 26 percent relative risk reduction (3.5 percent is approximately 26 percent of 13 percent), which misleads both patients and doctors because it exaggerates the benefits.

In the summary report, the authors were very keen to state that increasing the dose of the statin derived "incremental benefit." They also claimed that the study provided evidence for more intensive lowering of LDL "cholesterol" with statins for people with heart disease and metabolic syndrome. However, they failed to mention that even in this very high-risk group, increasing the dose of the statin to 80 mg did not make much difference in the total number of deaths, since 6.3 percent of the people in the 10 mg group died of all causes, compared with 6.2 percent in the 80 mg group. Although increasing the dose of the statin lowered LDL levels significantly more than the lower dosage, it also accompanied more deaths from noncardiovascular causes. The reduction in cardiovascular risk was almost completely countered by the increase in the risk of death from other causes. This study shows that lowering LDLs more intensively will not significantly increase life expectancy, even for people who are already at very high risk.

The WOSCOPS Study

The WOSCOPS study included 6,595 men from the western area of Scotland who had high cholesterol levels.[9] The average total cholesterol level for the men included in this study was 270 mg/dL (7.0 mmol/L). The WOSCOPS study has been used to justify the use of statins in the wider general population. The supporters of the cholesterol hypothesis have created an impression that having higher-than-average cholesterol drastically increases the risk of dying from heart disease. However, during this five-year study, 1.7 percent of men who were given the placebo died of heart disease, compared with 1.2 percent of those who were given the statin. It is also worth noting that overall, the use of the statin only increased a participant's chances of still being alive after five years from 96 percent to 97 percent.[10,11]

One interesting feature of the WOSCOPS study was that around 80 percent of the men included were current smokers or ex-smokers. It is well-known that smoking drastically increases the risk of heart disease. In fact, the heart disease death rate is 80 percent higher in heavy smokers than in nonsmokers.[12] We also know that smoking causes inflammation, and that this inflammation can take five years to reduce to normal levels after one stops smoking.[13] Heart disease is an inflammatory condition and statins reduce inflammation. Therefore, any benefits that were achieved in this trial could be due to the effect the statin had on inflammation, and possibly could have nothing to do with cholesterol. Further evidence that any benefits found in the WOSCOPS study might have had nothing to do with cholesterol is the fact that the men in the higher band of total cholesterol level benefited less than those in the lower band. This was also the case for the level of LDLs.

THE WOSCOPS FOLLOW-UP

After the initial WOSCOPS trial was completed, researchers undertook a ten-year follow up of the trial participants,[14] which was published in the *New England Journal of Medicine,* one of the most prestigious medical journals in the world. However, the follow-up study had a number of serious problems.

After the WOSCOPS trial, some of the participants from the placebo group started taking a statin, while some of those who were in the statin group stopped taking it. The researchers did not take into account that the original groups were mixed up in the WOSCOPS follow-up study, which should render any results obtained after ten years meaningless. To make matters worse, the researchers did not know how many people were taking statins for the full ten years; they only had data on this aspect from the first five years.

These important issues aside, the results of the study were (after the five-year period of the original WOSCOPS trial plus the ten-year follow-up period, a total of fifteen years) that 5.1 percent of the people who were originally given the statin had died of heart disease, compared with 6.3 percent in the original placebo group.

Interestingly, more people from the original statin group were diagnosed with cancer than from the original placebo group, though the authors of the study dismissed this as a chance finding. Favorable results for the statin were overemphasized, and negative results were dismissed as unimportant or chance findings. The effects that the statin had on the incidence of cancer in this study might be important because the fifteen-year study period is unusual for statin clinical trials, which are typically about five years in duration or less, and cancer does not usually appear after just five years; it can take decades to develop. The data from the WOSCOPS follow-up period actually shows that with increasing time, people who were in the original statin group had a higher incidence of cancer.

An editorial accompanying this study was also published in the *New England Journal of Medicine,*[15] in which the author stated that "there should no longer be any doubt that the reduction of LDL cholesterol levels has a role in the prevention and treatment of coronary heart disease." *The Times* newspaper also featured this study in an article that took up its entire front page, which suggested that "statins have benefits after dosage is stopped" and that statins should be used for even more people, "including younger people in whom heart disease has yet to get a start."[1] This is an example of how a poorly designed study can be translated into misleading information given to the general public. The WOSCOPS follow-up did not reveal anything new about statins other than their potential to increase the risk for cancer, yet the results were published in a way that proved to show statins in a highly favorable light.

Overall Analysis

The discussion above is intended to provide a flavor of the clinical trial data for statins, including studies that have been positive for statins, those that were negative, and examples of how the data is often misrepresented. However, in order to make sense of the data overall, it is necessary to separate it into two broad groups: primary prevention (those people who do not have a heart problem) and secondary prevention (those people with an existing heart problem).

Analysis of the primary prevention clinical trial data shows that there is no net benefit associated with the use of a statin for prevention. This is extremely important because at least 75 percent of all the people who currently take a statin are taking it for primary prevention.

In 2010, a meta-analysis of eleven statin trials was published in the *Archives of Internal Medicine*, in which Professor Kausik Ray and colleagues concluded that, when they are used in primary prevention, statins provide no net benefit in terms of deaths from all causes.[16]

This analysis had the cleanest dataset of any analysis completed to date; the researchers were able to exclude patients with existing heart disease (secondary prevention) and only include data associated with primary prevention.

In 2011, the Cochrane Collaboration conducted a review of statin clinical trials. After this review, lead authors Dr. Shah Ebrahim and Dr. Fiona Taylor said that they could not recommend the use of statins for primary prevention.* The absolute benefit was so small that it could have been down to chance, and even if it were a real benefit, 1,000 people would have to be treated for one year to prevent one death.[17]

Despite these negative findings, both pharmaceutical companies and health authorities have continued to relentlessly forge ahead to put more and more people onto statins.

Another way to look at the overall data for primary prevention is to use the number needed to treat (NNT). This number is commonly used for evaluating the benefits versus risks associated with a medication. The NNT equals the number of people that would have to be treated in order to see an effect.

The NNT for the use of statins in primary prevention[18] is as follows:

- No lives saved (no extension of life expectancy)
- 1 heart attack prevented per 60 people treated
- 1 stroke prevented per 268 people treated

---

* It should be mentioned that the Cochrane group updated their review in 2013 and at that time changed their recommendation in favor of the widespread use of statins. This is discussed in considerable detail in *Statin Nation II: What Really Causes Heart Disease?* Suffice it to say that this second review included work done by a research group who refuse to release their data for public scrutiny; the group maintains that the data is commercially sensitive.

- 1 person will develop diabetes per 50 people treated
- 1 person will suffer muscle damage per 10 people treated

Clearly, the data for primary prevention shows that people do not live any longer when taking a statin; however, contrary to what we are told, significant numbers of people are affected by side effects. In addition, this NNT analysis did not include additional side effects that have since come to light, such as: damage to the eyes, kidney disease, and deterioration of brain function, as we shall see when we discuss statin side effects, below.

What about secondary prevention? As we have seen, some of the secondary prevention clinical trials have shown a modest reduction in deaths from all causes, typically a 1 percent or 2 percent reduction in the mortality rate. Although this is not a huge reduction in risk, 1 percent or 2 percent applied across a population equals millions of people. If the side effects of statins were mild and very rare, then the use of statins in secondary prevention could be worthwhile.

Statins do have some beneficial effects for patients with heart problems. The exact mechanisms are still being debated; however, it appears that statins can help stabilize arterial plaques, reduce inflammation, and improve iron metabolism, which in turn might also prevent progression and destabilization of atherosclerotic plaque.[19]

On the other hand, statins have also been shown to be bad for the heart. Statins block the normal adapting process that enables the heart to recover and strengthen in response to physical exercise. Statins can also, somewhat paradoxically, increase the amount of calcified plaque in the arteries. And statins weaken the heart by blocking coenzyme Q10. Statins also block vitamin K_2 and selenium containing proteins, which are also important for proper heart function.[20] In addition, the lowering of cholesterol itself is strongly associated with a reduced life expectancy because low cholesterol is associated with liver disease, cancer, and serious infections.[21]

Estimates suggest that around 100 million people are currently taking a statin, and statins are intended to be taken for decades. For a medication that is so widely prescribed and used for such a long period of time, the question of their efficacy must be answered in terms of any improvement in life expectancy. And if statins do improve life expectancy, is it enough to offset the chance of side effects? A recent analysis published in the *British Medical Journal* could serve to answer this question. When researchers analyzed data from statin clinical trials that reported on deaths from all causes and estimated the average life extension that could be expected from taking a statin in both primary and secondary prevention,[22] the results suggested that in primary prevention an average life extension of 3.2 days could be expected, and 4.1 days in secondary prevention.

Statin Side Effects

The most common side effects of cholesterol-lowering statins are, perhaps unsurprisingly, directly related to the parts of the body that we know require more cholesterol. The brain and nervous system, immune system, eyes, and cellular membranes all require large amounts of cholesterol in order to function properly. In addition, cholesterol is the raw material for the production of all of the steroidal hormones, vitamin D, and bile acids for digestion. Therefore, when the production of cholesterol is blocked by a statin, these systems, organs, and processes often suffer first. However, because of the way that statins work, they hinder the production of a number of other essential life-sustaining molecules.

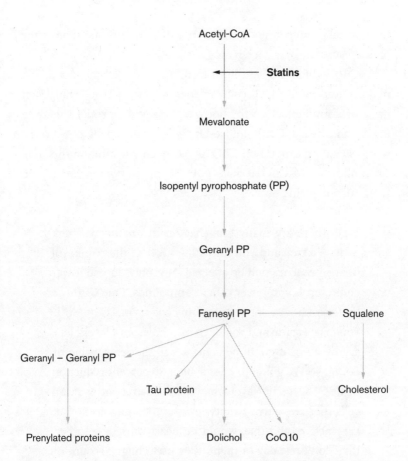

Figure 4.1. The mevalonate pathway and the action of statins.

Statins act very high up in the mevalonate pathway, a complex sequence of biochemical reactions that naturally occur in all cells for the production of cholesterol and many other essential molecules. The mevalonate pathway can be represented as a tree diagram, as shown in figure 4.1.

Statins block an enzyme near the top of this tree, which effectively also blocks the downstream biochemical reactions, including

the normal production of a wide range of biochemicals. One of the
blocked substances is coenzyme Q10 (CoQ10).

CoQ10, which we'll explore in more depth in chapter 6, is a
major component of all cellular energy; reducing its availability
has a profound effect on the body, especially the proper functioning of the heart. Cardiologist Dr. Peter Langsjoen, one of the
world's leading experts on CoQ10, has been working on the clinical application of CoQ10 since 1983. In the film *Statin Nation*, Dr.
Langsjoen explains:

> Well, there are many branches on this pathway; think
> of it as a tree and you're cutting it off at the trunk: All
> of the branches will be affected. Not only do you lower
> cholesterol, you lower other compounds. One of those
> that we know a lot about is this coenzyme Q10. So if
> you take a statin and you decrease cholesterol levels, let's
> say by 40 or even 50 percent, which they're capable of
> doing, you're going to have a 40 or 50 percent reduction
> in CoQ10. It's not avoidable; it's the same pathway. So
> cells that are active twenty-four hours a day every day,
> very active, and that would be heart muscle cells . . .
> they don't rest day or night, they use a huge amount of
> energy. And therefore heart muscle has the highest con-
> centration of CoQ10, by far.

The unfortunate and somewhat paradoxical effect of taking
a statin to reduce cholesterol, therefore, is that it blocks the production of one of the most important molecules for the function
of the heart. Statins also further reduce the availability of CoQ10
because CoQ10 is carried through the bloodstream as part of the
LDL particles, the transport mechanism for delivering CoQ10 to the

cells where it is needed. LDLs also provide the transport mechanism for a number of other vital nutrients such as vitamin E, and various carotenoids such as beta-carotene.[23,24]

CoQ10, vitamin E, beta-carotene, and other carotenoids are all antioxidants, which are important to the body because they stabilize free radicals. Free radicals are a normal part of our biology; however, when they are out of control they can accelerate the aging process, cause complications with diabetes, and contribute to a range of other disorders. The main process by which free radicals do damage is related to the normal action of oxidation whereby molecules lose an electron. Antioxidants, such as CoQ10, vitamin E, and beta-carotene serve as electron donors and deactivate the free radicals, preventing them from injuring cells. Vitamin E, in addition to being an antioxidant, plays a number of other very important roles within the body, including:

- Ensuring proper functioning of the circulatory system, nervous system, digestive system, excretory system, and respiratory system
- Helping to maintain the integrity of cell membranes, including red blood cells, nerve cells, kidney tissues, the lungs, and the liver
- Promoting normal growth patterns and the body's ability to respond to stress
- Stimulating proper development and tone of the skeletal muscles, the heart, and the intestines[25,26]

Low blood levels of vitamin E could be associated with disorders of the central nervous system, deterioration of the brain, and progression to Alzheimer's disease. A low blood level of vitamin E is also predictive of heart disease.[27]

Statin manufacturers would have us believe that side effects related to statins are rare and are mild when they do occur. Statin supporters quote data from selected clinical trials that have reported a low rate of side effects. Unfortunately, the reality is very different. Populations selected for clinical trials are chosen very carefully and are often very different from real-life population groups. Researchers carefully screen people for existing medical conditions when recruiting participants, and they exclude many on the basis of being of childbearing age (if female) and having a history of drug or alcohol abuse, poor mental function, heart failure, arrhythmia and other heart conditions, liver and kidney disorders, cancer, other serious diseases, and hypersensitivity to statins. Candidates to whom any of the above applies are routinely excluded from such trials.

In addition, clinical trials often have a run-in period where even more people can be excluded. Participants typically take the drug in question for a few weeks, and if they experience any adverse effects or if they decide not to continue for any other reason, they are withdrawn from the trial. All of this means that the people who finally make it into the actual clinical trial are precisely chosen and are no longer representative of the general population. Consider one trial conducted to evaluate a new drug aimed at increasing good cholesterols (HDLs). Of the 19,000 people assessed for eligibility, more than 2,000 were excluded before the run-in phase, and almost another 2,000 were excluded before the trial officially started.[28,29] It might well be the case that some of these people were excluded for safety reasons; however, questions remain concerning how many of the people excluded would ordinarily be prescribed statins outside of the trial.

Around half of all statin clinical trials to date have failed to report on side effects, and necessary post-marketing drug surveillance, where drugs are approved on the condition that further data will be collected after the drug has entered the market, is not always performed.[30] This post-marketing evaluation is critical, as was highlighted in the case of cerivastatin, which was withdrawn from use in 2001 after it was linked to the deaths of 52 patients.[31] More than 10 percent of approved drugs are subsequently required to include one or more prominent black box safety warnings (which are added to the packaging of the drug and indicate that there might be very serious or life-threatening adverse effects) or are withdrawn from the market completely.[30]

Despite the importance of post-marketing surveillance, more than half of the studies pharmaceutical companies promise to conduct once their drug is released into the marketplace are not completed.[32] Many adverse effects are first recognized by post-marketing surveillance, and the rate of adverse effects is likely to be higher than we think because doctors often do not report them.[33] In addition, pharmaceutical companies might selectively publish only results that are favorable to their drug, leading to bias and misrepresentation of the totality of the data.

Dr. Malcolm Kendrick, writing in the *British Medical Journal* about the adverse effects of statins,[34] explains that definitive evidence for the severity of statin adverse effects comes from the US FDA adverse event reporting system, which showed that between 1997 and 2004 one statin (simvastatin) was reported as a direct cause of 49,350 adverse events and 416 deaths. Since adverse events are greatly underreported, the actual figures are likely to be much higher.[35]

Statins and Cancer

Statin manufacturers are very keen to quote clinical trials that show their drugs do not lead to an increased incidence of cancer.

However, most statin trials last just a few years, while cancer normally takes decades to develop. For example, smokers do not usually get cancer within the first few years after taking up their first cigarette. If statins do increase the risk for cancer, then it should be seen first in groups of people at high risk, such as the elderly.[33] The PROSPER trial tested the effects of statins on older people (aged seventy to eighty-two years)[36] and found more frequent cancer diagnoses in people who took the statin compared with those who did not. The risk of heart disease was slightly reduced, but this was countered by an increased risk of cancer associated with the statin after just three years of follow-up. A study published in the *Journal of the American College of Cardiology* also found that any cardiovascular benefits were offset by an increased risk of cancer.[34] For an in-depth discussion of statins and cancer, readers are referred to an excellent open access article by Dr. Ravnskov, Dr. McCully, and Professor Rosch.[37]

Psychological and Nervous System Problems

Cholesterol is vital for the development and function of the brain. It is therefore unsurprising that mental and neurological complaints have often been observed when cholesterol levels are reduced.[33] Duane Graveline, a former astronaut, aerospace medical research scientist, flight surgeon, and family doctor, a person with obvious considerable intellectual and physical agility, is not the sort of person you would expect to find wandering aimlessly in the woods and unable to recognize his own wife. Yet this is exactly what happened to him after taking the statin Lipitor. After taking the drug for just six weeks, Dr. Graveline experienced transient global amnesia (TGA), a sudden episode of memory loss.

Amnesia was not listed as a side effect of statins, but Dr. Graveline suspected the drug as the cause since it was a new medicine for him and he had not experienced any of these symptoms prior to taking it. For one year Dr. Graveline stopped taking Lipitor, in which he had no reoccurrence of the amnesia. Then, after his next astronaut physical, his NASA doctors suggested he started taking the drug again. After six weeks of being back on Lipitor he had his second attack of TGA.

After his experiences, Dr. Graveline further investigated the link between statins and memory loss. He found hundreds of case reports from patients, relatives, and even doctors describing a full array of cognitive side effects, from amnesia and severe memory loss to confusion and disorientation, all associated with the use of statins.[38]

Studies within the scientific literature provide further evidence of a link between statins and cognitive impairment.[39,40] One study, for example, found that the use of statins was associated with manifestations of severe irritability, homicidal impulses, threats to others, road rage, fear of family members, and damage to property. In each case the personality disruption was sustained until the statin was stopped.[41]

In 2012, researchers at the University of Arizona screened a large number of medications for possible adverse effects on nerve cells, with tests performed on fruit flies.[42] Normally, a great deal of caution should be applied when attempting to extrapolate what is seen in animal studies to effects in humans; however, this study raised a shocking possibility of which more people should be aware. The researchers tested 1,040 different compounds. Of these, only four compounds created bead-like growths within the nerve cells, bead-like growths that would hinder nerve transmission. All four of the compounds that caused this effect were statins.

Studies have shown that statins can also cause erectile dysfunction[43] and a reduction in libido,[44] probably mediated through low testosterone levels (statins block the production of all of the sex hormones).[44]

Muscle Pain, Weakness, and Rhabdomyolysis

All statin drugs have been associated with diseases of the muscles. The most common adverse effects reported are general muscle pain or weakness; however, this can in rare cases lead to rhabdomyolysis.[33,45] Rhabdomyolysis is the breakdown of muscle resulting in the release of muscle fiber contents (myoglobin) into the bloodstream, which is harmful to the kidney and sometimes fatal. However, it is extremely difficult to establish the incidence of muscle-related problems among people who take statins. Muscle pain and fatigue often go undetected[44] and are often wrongly assumed to be age-related. Muscle problems become worse the higher the statin dose,[46] and there are additional concerns when other medications are taken at the same time.[47] Level of dosage is an important consideration because it has been suggested that some people take higher doses of statins in order to reduce LDL levels more.[48]

Exercise also seems to exacerbate symptoms of muscle pain and weakness.[49–51] A person taking statins will be less likely to exercise if it causes pain and discomfort, and therefore will not be able to make appropriate lifestyle changes in order to reduce their risk of a heart attack.

Muscle pain and weakness are often downplayed as minor adverse effects; patients are even sometimes expected to live with the pain in order to "benefit" from the statin. In reality, thousands of people have had their lives ruined by statin muscle damage. In a percentage of cases the damage is permanent.

Diabetes

It is now widely acknowledged that statins cause type 2 diabetes (T2DM), as acknowledged by the US FDA, which lists T2DM as a side effect. This is likely due to the effects that statins have on steroidal hormone balance.

Eye Problems

The lens of the eye requires a large amount of cholesterol; therefore, cholesterol-lowering statins increase the risk for cataracts. The cataracts caused by statins are sometimes severe enough to warrant surgery.[51]

Heart Disease

Atherosclerosis is a hardening and narrowing of the arteries, a process that involves calcification. Statins increase the calcification of the arteries. The CONFIRM (COronary CT Angiography EvaluatioN For Clinical Outcomes: An InteRnational Multicenter) registry found that statin use is associated with an increased number and extent of calcified coronary plaques,[52] which is ironic for a drug that is marketed to lower the risk of cardiovascular disease. Other studies have shown that statins do not reduce coronary artery calcium, and that the disease continues regardless of the statin.[53,54]

The Veteran Affairs Diabetes Trial[55] found that statin use was linked with the progression of coronary artery calcification in people with T2DM without previous coronary artery disease, despite the fact that the statin users had significantly lower and nearly optimal LDL cholesterol levels.

Statins probably increase the amount of calcified plaque in the arteries because of statin inhibition of vitamin K_2 and selenium, both of which normally have a protective effect.

Statins have another detrimental effect on the heart. Consider that when we exercise, the heart gets stronger. This adaptation to exercise is important for everyone, and in particular, it is an important part of the recovery process for cardiac patients. Exercise stimulates

the body to make more mitochondria, the energy-producing factories within muscle cells. However, statins have been found to block
this adaptation.[56] This is one of the many side effects that are conveniently ignored when statins are prescribed.

CHAPTER FIVE

The Real Causes of Heart Disease

The previous chapters examined the scientific basis for the diet-heart hypothesis, the benefits and risks associated with statins, and the argument that cholesterol is not the cause of heart disease. So if not cholesterol, what *does* cause heart disease? This chapter covers the many causes currently overlooked due to the disproportionate attention given to cholesterol.

Hearts and Minds

The biggest oversight in both the current model of heart disease and cardiovascular risk calculators is that they do not consider the impact of stress. Psychological and physical stress are two of the most important causes of heart disease and heart attacks, yet health authorities barely even consider stress. Some health authorities even categorically state that stress is *not* important,[1] which demonstrates how unfit for purpose some health authorities have become where heart disease is concerned.

Stress directly affects the condition of the arteries, the likelihood that blood clots will form, the health of the heart muscle itself, and the electrical system that controls the heart. Stress also "burns up" essential nutrients that would otherwise protect us from heart disease. And stress weakens the immune system such that we can become more vulnerable to infections, which could also play a role in the development of heart disease. But before discussing these stress effects, let's briefly discuss a few subtle points about what stress actually is.

One of the key characteristics of stress is that it is an individual phenomenon. What one person finds stressful, another person can find enjoyably stimulating. For example, some people thrive when asked to give a public or professional presentation; they accept every invitation for public speaking and thoroughly enjoy the experience. Other people are filled with complete horror at the thought of standing up in front of an audience for even a moment. Similarly, some people thrive in unpredictable circumstances. This type of person's occupation might be one where no two days are the same; each day is full of unexpected challenges. Although this might seem stressful to some people, others find it stimulating, and it has a positive effect on their well-being. However, if someone who thrives in an unpredictable environment is forced into a predictable unchanging situation, they, too, will become stressed. In addition, some people seem to be able to cope with more negative stress than others through a greater capacity to deal with a particular stressor, and excess negative stress manifests as different symptom profiles for different people.

Aside from the individual differences in what people experience as stressful, is the perception of stress itself, which is what determines if an event or situation (a potential stressor) will harm us or not. To understand the importance of this fact we have to understand the basic stress response.

A full description of the stress response involves an encyclopedic amount of medical terminology; however, the key stages in the

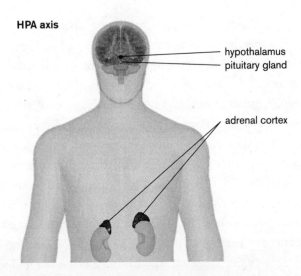

HPA axis

hypothalamus
pituitary gland

adrenal cortex

Figure 5.1. Anatomical positions of the hypothalamus, pituitary, and adrenal glands (the HPA axis). Image courtesy Anatomography/Wikimedia Commons.

process are readily appreciable. The process starts with the perception of stress. The brain makes a decision about whether a situation is stressful or not, based on sensory input (principally what we see and hear) and on stored memory (recalling what happened the last time a similar situation occurred). If the brain decides that the situation is stressful, the hypothalamus (located at the base of the brain) triggers the stress response, sending a signal to the pituitary gland (also at the base of the brain), which in turn sends a signal to the adrenal glands. The adrenal glands then release into the body several hormones, such as cortisol, adrenaline (epinephrine), and noradrenaline (norepinephrine), in order to help the body deal with the stressor. Technically this is known as the hypothalamic-pituitary-adrenal axis, or HPA axis. The positions of the various glands are shown in figure 5.1.

The HPA axis works closely with the autonomic nervous system (ANS), which controls everything in the body that works automatically. There are two branches of the ANS: the parasympathetic branch switches on body functions associated with rest, repair, and recovery, and also slows the heart rate, whereas the sympathetic branch increases the heart rate and enables the body to take action when needed, either to run quickly from a stressor or attacker, or to change the body's physiology in order to fight the stressor or attacker.

The stress response is designed to cope with a physical threat. Our ancestors, when faced with a physical threat, had to flee or fight. Therefore, in the face of a threat, the sympathetic nervous system prepares the body for this by increasing the heart rate, making the blood easier to coagulate (in the case of an injury the blood must be able to easily clot in order to minimize blood loss), increasing circulation to the working muscles, and making glucose (a rapid source of energy) available.

At the same time, the parasympathetic nervous system is down-regulated. After all, in the face of an immediate threat, there is not sufficient time to digest food and perform repair functions. The assimilation of nutrients and general rest and repair can be taken care of later. In the face of an immediate threat, only the sympathetic nervous system is needed to get us out of immediate danger.

In simple terms, the sympathetic and parasympathetic systems can be thought of as having opposite functions, as illustrated in table 5.1, which shows how some major organs and functions of the body are affected by each branch of the autonomic nervous system.

Stressors that affect people in the twenty-first century do not usually require that we run away or fight. Usually modern stressors require a creative or logical solution, rather than an instinctive reaction. So, in some ways, the body's stress response is out of date. And this has important considerations for heart disease.

For example, today it is common for one's stress response to be continuously activated without an adequate resolution to

Table 5.1. Main Actions of the Parasympathetic and Sympathetic Branches of the Autonomic Nervous System

Parasympathetic	Sympathetic
oonotrioto pupilo	dilatoo pupilo
increases saliva production	inhibits saliva production
reduces the heart rate	increases the heart rate
constricts bronchia	dilates bronchia
stimulates digestion activity	inhibits digestion activity
stimulates pancreatic activity	inhibits pancreatic activity
stimulates the gallbladder	inhibits the gallbladder
	stimulates adrenal glands to release adrenaline and noradrenaline
constricts urinary bladder	relaxes urinary bladder
stimulates erection of genitals	stimulates orgasm in genitals

the stressor. The stress response is designed to cope with shorter immediate threat–type situations, but an inappropriate working environment, an abusive relationship, financial hardship, or a lack of social support often become chronic situations that continuously activate the stress response with little opportunity for the repair functions of the parasympathetic system to be fully activated.

The result can be a continuously down-regulated parasympathetic system and an over-activated sympathetic system, a state that has been referred to as tired and wired. If nothing changes to relieve the chronic stressors, a state of exhaustion eventually sets in where the body can no longer provide an adequate stress response and even minor stressors begin to have a major impact on the body. At this stage many of the normal bodily adaptations that keep us healthy on a daily basis stop working efficiently.

Types of Stressful Situations

As mentioned, stress is a highly individual phenomenon. It is universally acknowledged that a certain amount of stress can be beneficial
and can be associated with an increase in productivity and performance. However, there is a point at which the stress becomes too
much and performance starts to deteriorate. When performance
deteriorates, health deteriorates, and exhaustion eventually results
if the stressor, or stressors, are not managed.

Though it might be obvious, it is worth mentioning that stress
can come from a wide range of different psychological and physical stressors. Most people are familiar with the stress associated
with academic or professional examinations, a work-related project
deadline, managing multiple projects, or writing a book. During
the process of completing these tasks we can at times feel quite
terrible. We might even start to exhibit some temporary symptoms
associated with stress, such as insomnia, stomach complaints, or
a general loss of energy and vitality. However, thankfully, there
is usually a resolution to these types of stressful situations. The
project will eventually be completed, the exams undertaken, the
book written. This, we hope, leads to a successful conclusion that
provides an opportunity for the sympathetic nervous system to be
calmed and the parasympathetic nervous system to begin repair
and recovery.

Stress research suggests that the most damaging forms of psychological stress are associated with chronic unrelenting situations,
such as feeling a lack of control over one's personal circumstances
or having prolonged financial worries, a lack of social support, and
posttraumatic stress.

Different socioeconomic groups have dramatically different levels
of health. This is particularly the case where heart disease is concerned. People in the lowest socioeconomic group are up to five

times more likely to die of heart disease than people in the highest socioeconomic group, despite having similar cholesterol levels.[2-5] Nutritional status and other factors might play a role, but this dramatic difference in heart disease mortality can only be explained by looking at the psychological impact that different environments and life circumstances produce.

Additional data suggesting that certain types of psychological stress are particularly damaging comes from the Whitehall Study, a long-running landmark study of civil servants in England.[6] Striking differences in health corresponded with levels of seniority within the civil service. The higher up a person was within the civil service hierarchy, the less likely he or she was to suffer health problems, particularly cardiovascular health–related problems. The health risks correlated with the degree of control a person felt he or she had within a position; the more control the person felt, the less likely he or she was to suffer heart problems.

Another important finding from the Whitehall Study relates to the effort/reward ratio. Those people reporting a low effort with high reward had a significantly lower heart disease risk than those people reporting a high effort with little reward.

Stress can also come from physical sources such as injury and pain. In fact, any medical condition is associated with both physical and mental stress. And, in general, all of the stressful factors accumulate toward the overall stress load upon the mind and body.

Physiological Changes Caused by Stress

During the downward spiral toward exhaustion, a number of physiological changes occur that increase the risk for heart disease. The activation of both the stress response and the sympathetic nervous system causes the release of adrenaline (epinephrine) and cortisol. These hormones have many effects. Adrenaline makes the blood more readily able to clot in the case of a physical injury. As we already know, blood clots are an important feature of heart disease.

Adrenaline also affects the heart rate and blood vessels so that cardiac output increases (increasing circulation to the working muscles), increasing blood pressure. Increased blood pressure could increase the risk of damage to the inside wall of the arteries and, hence, contribute to heart disease risk. The increase in blood pressure is only temporary; normal blood pressure is restored once the stress response has been deactivated. However, as mentioned in the previous section, many people today are experiencing a chronic activation of the stress response.

The hormone cortisol has the effect of raising blood glucose levels. Cortisol also contributes to obesity, in particular, central obesity (visceral fat), which has been identified as the more dangerous type of obesity.[7] Overall, changes in blood glucose, increased central obesity, increased blood pressure, and other metabolic changes can increase the risk for type 2 diabetes (T2DM), and people who have T2DM have up to five times the risk of developing heart disease compared to people who don't have T2DM.

Cortisol has a weakening effect on the immune system, which is one reason why people who are chronically stressed often become more susceptible to infections. Infections could also play a role in heart disease. Cortisol also prevents the body's cells from losing sodium and encourages the cellular loss of potassium. This imbalance could lead to fluid retention and dysfunction of the cell to the extent that it contributes to heart muscle cell death.

Major stressors can cause a heart attack directly without any existing damage to the arteries or any other risk factors, due to the effects of noradrenaline (norepinephrine), which is also released during the stress response. Noradrenaline is released to enable stronger muscle contractions. It is released at nerve endings and can cause bands of cell death (technically known as contraction band necrosis).

Stress encourages us to eat poor quality foods and miss out on important heart protective nutrients, as well as to consume more sugar, drink more alcohol, and smoke cigarettes. All of these poor lifestyle choices also impact the balance of the autonomic nervous system, making things worse. In particular, smoking cigarettes further activates the sympathetic nervous system.

Stress also causes takotsubo cardiomyopathy, also known as broken-heart syndrome, which is a weakening of the heart's main pumping chamber as a result of severe emotional or physical stress.

However, this is just the tip of the iceberg where stress and its effects on the heart via the autonomic nervous system are concerned. Even more profound and significant are the changes in heart rate variability and the acidity of the heart.

Heart Rate Variability

We have already seen how the body's stress response is activated through the parasympathetic and sympathetic nervous system: a down regulating of the parasympathetic system and an up regulating of the sympathetic system. Another way of looking at the activity of the parasympathetic system is by measuring vagal tone.

The parasympathetic system is activated through the vagus nerve, which originates from the base of the brain. A decrease in vagal activity, by definition, is the same as a decrease in parasympathetic nervous activity. A number of studies have shown that heart disease is associated with a reduction in vagal activity.[8–18] It is conceivable that the reduction in vagal activity is a result of heart disease rather than the cause, bringing us back to the chicken-and-egg scenario mentioned in chapter 1. However, studies have also shown that the disease process within the arteries cannot account for the totality of the decrease in vagal activity.[13,18–21]

In fact, vagal activity is actually measured through heart rate variability (HRV); vagal tone cannot be measured directly. HRV represents the activity of the vagus nerve and is an accurate alternative biological measurement since an increase in vagal tone (parasympathetic nervous system activity) slows the heart rate down and an increase in sympathetic nervous system activity speeds it up.

HRV refers to the difference in the time interval between beats of the heart. If the time interval between beats varies a lot, there is a high HRV. One might assume that a predictable, uniform heartbeat (low HRV) is healthy, but in fact the reverse is true. A healthy heart displays a high degree of variability in the beat-to-beat time intervals, as the heart adjusts to whatever demands are placed upon it.

Increased HRV reflects increased vagal tone and hence increased parasympathetic activity, while reduced HRV has been shown to predict heart disease death, as well as deaths from all causes.[22–26]

One study published in the *Journal of the American College of Cardiology* in 2001 followed participants for ten years and found that reduced HRV was associated with more than four times the risk of sudden cardiac death.[24] The researchers cited excessive sympathetic nervous system activation as the likely cause of the impairment.

Another study published in the same journal the same year found that HRV drops even further immediately before a heart attack,[27] noting a gradual decline in HRV starting one hour before a heart attack occurred. The decrease in HRV was even more obvious two minutes before a heart attack, and during the heart attack event itself there was an almost complete withdrawal of vagal activity. The decrease in HRV and the corresponding heart attack were also more closely related to activities associated with mental stress, confirming the results of earlier studies that suggested a link between reduced parasympathetic activity, mental stress, and heart attacks.[28] And, according to another study, the end of the heart attack event itself coincides with the recurrence of vagal activity.[29]

Acidosis

The activation of the stress response, the withdrawal of the parasympathetic nervous system, and the release of adrenaline (epinephrine) cause the heart to change the way it produces energy. The heart prefers to use fat for its main source of energy (a fact which is a contradiction of sixty years' worth of health advice suggesting that dietary fat is bad for the heart).[30] However, the release of adrenaline as a result of the stress response causes the heart to use the glucose-burning energy system instead of the preferred fat-burning energy system.

The fat-burning energy system yields more energy, but it involves a slower process. When you consider that the stress response is designed to help us flee from danger or fight an attacker, it is not surprising that the stress response causes a shift to glucose metabolism; the glucose-burning energy system makes energy available more quickly, though at a cost: rapid production of lactic acid.

All athletes are aware of the effects of lactic acid. When undertaking strenuous exercise, lactic acid builds up in the muscles as a kind of metabolic by-product. If lactic acid builds up more quickly than the body can remove it, a burning sensation is felt in the working muscles. Eventually, the lactic acid causes muscle fatigue and reduces the ability of the muscles to contract, slowing down performance.

The heart's temporary shift to burning glucose as part of the stress response probably worked well for our ancestors, enabling them to deal with immediate threats. However, repeated or chronic activation of the stress response can cause a significant change in the biochemistry of the heart, whereby the heart muscle becomes more

acidic.[29,31] Acidosis blocks the ability of calcium ions to activate contraction.[32] This results in an impairment of blood supply to heart
muscle cells, leading to cell death (a heart attack).[29]

Acidosis, combined with other aspects of the stress response,
could also cause vascular stretching that leads to damage to the
inside wall of the arteries. Acidosis could cause blood vessels to
dilate, while at the same time, the activation of the sympathetic nervous system causes blood vessels to constrict.[33] This simultaneous
pulling and pushing on the vessels could cause vascular stretching
and alter the shear stress within the arteries. This change in fluid
dynamics could be in addition to changes in blood flow as a result of
the damaged heart muscle tissue.

Some researchers have stated that biomechanical stress is the
most important cause of damage to the inside wall of the arteries.[34]
Once this damage occurs, a blood clot forms within the artery and
the repair processes are called into action. If damage occurs repeatedly, then other substances, such as white blood cells, cholesterol,
and other molecules, are sent to the site of damage in order to deal
with the problem. The combination of substances that are then
contained within the wall of the artery form a plaque, causing the
characteristic coronary artery disease.

Researchers have known about the acidosis theory of heart
attacks for some time. Writing for the *British Heart Journal* in 1971,
Dr. L. H. Opie, from the Medical Research Council's cardiovascular
unit in London, once opined, "It is sobering to recall that many of
the important metabolic changes in experimental myocardial infarction [heart attacks] have been known for over thirty years."[35] Indeed,
research papers describing acidosis of the heart and how it relates to
heart attacks go back as far as 1925.[36,37]

In case there is any remaining doubt about stress as a primary
cause of heart attacks and death, a study published in the journal

Circulation in 2012 investigated the use of transcendental meditation for people with heart disease.[38] Participants were split into two groups; one group completed twenty minutes of meditation twice every day, while the other, dubbed the "health education group," was instructed to spend the same amount of time doing other health-promoting activities such as preparing healthy meals, exercising, or nonspecific relaxation.

After five years of follow-up, 31 percent of the people in the health education group had either had a heart attack or stroke, or died, compared with 20 percent of those in the meditation group, representing an absolute risk reduction of 11 percent associated with meditation, above the benefits associated with more common health-promoting activities.

This study was a secondary prevention trial, which means its participants already had a diagnosis of heart disease at the start of the study. Secondary prevention trials done on statins have shown that statins typically reduce the risk of heart attack and death from all causes by about 1 percent or 2 percent,[2,39] the exception being the 4S Study completed in 1994, which found an absolute risk reduction in all-cause mortality of around 4 percent. No other clinical trial done on statins since has come anywhere close to the 4S's level of risk reduction.[40]

The data suggests that meditation for twenty minutes twice each day is between five and eleven times more beneficial than taking a statin (depending on which statin clinical trial we use for comparison). Still, leading health authorities maintain that stress is not a cause of heart disease, and there are no public health incentives to encourage stress management.

It is clear that excessive activation of the stress response causes heart disease and heart attacks, though this is currently ignored by many experts and health authorities, most likely as a result of the direct or subtle influence of the pharmaceutical industry.

The heart disease prevention plan in chapter 8 includes information about stress reduction. However, it is important to manage stress before reaching the exhaustion stage. Once a state of exhaustion has been reached, the situation becomes significantly more difficult to resolve. For example, chapter 7 discusses the importance of magnesium in heart disease. Magnesium is an incredibly important nutrient for the heart, and many people are undoubtedly magnesium-deficient, as we'll explore in chapter 7. However, magnesium supplements should not be taken in cases of a poor digestive system, and stress can weaken the digestive system. So, stress reduction should be a key fundamental aspect of everyone's heart disease prevention plan.

The Immune System

Microorganisms and spores enter the body through the airways, skin, and digestive system. The body often deals with these invaders by binding them to other substances in order to deactivate and remove them. In fact, LDL particles (the so-called bad cholesterol) participate in this process.[3] Major microbial invasions sometimes involve various particles sticking together to form aggregates, complexes consisting of larger bundles of substances involved in the immune response. These complexes are engulfed by a type of white blood cell called a macrophage.

When the immune system is working well, the contents of macrophages are destroyed and no harmful effects occur. However, if the immune system is compromised, these complexes could become trapped in the vasa vasorum of the arteries.[41]

The coronary arteries (along with the blood vessels that provide collateral circulation) supply blood and oxygen to the heart. But the walls of the coronary arteries are sufficiently large to require their own circulation. This is provided by the vasa vasorum, "the vessels of the vessels." The vasa vasorum consist of small branching vessels that retrieve some of the blood flowing through the arteries and send it into the artery wall itself. Because of the small size of the vasa vasorum, complexes containing microbes are more likely to get trapped, causing an obstruction in the vasa vasorum. This cuts off the supply of blood and oxygen to the arterial wall, leading to localized cell death within the artery wall.

When microorganisms and other contents of the complexes enter the area of dead tissue, more damage can occur. Eventually a microabscess is formed within the arterial wall, whose appearance will be the same, and contain the same substances, as the arterial plaque with which we are more familiar. If the abscess ruptures, the contents will be released into the artery, and the body will respond by forming a blood clot. If the blood clot completely blocks the artery, it might cause or contribute to a heart attack.

This theory of one of the pathways of heart attacks was proposed by Dr. Uffe Ravnskov, an independent researcher from Sweden who has published more than 150 articles that are critical of the cholesterol hypothesis, in many of the world's most respected medical journals.[42] Dr. Ravnskov is the author of the classic text *The Cholesterol Myths*,[43] which quite literally ignited the medical community. When it was first published in 2000, the book was deliberately set on fire during live television. Such was the challenge to the current dogma surrounding heart disease.

It is fair to say that Dr. Ravnskov's book prompted tens of thousands of researchers to reevaluate the causes of heart disease, and in turn those researchers have informed hundreds of thousands of people through their subsequent work. Dr. Ravnskov's work was central to informing people all around the world about the misinformation being perpetuated about cholesterol and saturated fat.

In 2009, Dr. Ravnskov, along with coauthor Dr. Kilmer McCully, published a detailed article explaining how infections and the immune system might contribute to the causes of heart disease.[44] After reviewing the medical literature, Drs. Ravnskov and McCully cited a number of intriguing findings, including:

- A high incidence of arterial damage in patients who died from typhoid fever[45]
- A connection between the degree of arterial plaque and the length of the preceding infection in people who had died from an infectious disease[46]
- An increase in cardiovascular deaths during influenza epidemics[47]
- An infectious disease immediately before a cardiovascular event in one third of heart attack and stroke patients[48]
- Dental problems due to infection and bacteremia (bacteria in the blood) associated with an increased risk of cardiovascular disease[49,50]

In addition, a large study published in 2016 found a strong correlation between a general marker for the immune system and heart disease.[51] Immunoglobulin G (IgG), a major antibody released in the presence of an invader, protects the body against bacterial and viral infections. People with higher levels of IgG were found to be protected against cardiovascular problems. The strongest connection was seen between high IgG levels and a lower incidence of heart disease. The lead researcher, Dr. Ramzi Khamis, consultant cardiologist and independent clinical research fellow at the National Heart and Lung Institute, Imperial College London, said, "Linking a stronger, more robust immune system to protection from heart attacks is a really exciting finding."[52]

However, factors associated with the immune system and heart disease cannot be considered in isolation. Dr. Ravnskov agrees that many other factors interact with the immune system,[33] stress in particular, since the stress response weakens the immune system. In addition, nutritional status, acidosis of the heart, the sodium/potassium balance, and environmental toxins also interact with the immune system and heart attack risk.

The immune system is another important aspect of heart disease that is currently completely ignored by the health authorities, the clinical guidelines, and the cardiovascular risk scores used by doctors.

Environmental Factors

A visit to the doctor to discuss cardiovascular risk is unlikely to include a discussion of the environment. Perhaps this is because there is no pill to manage the risks associated with the environment, but to be fair, the risks are difficult to pin down and many other factors intimately interrelate with environmental ones, including stress, lifestyle, nutrition, socioeconomic status, and others.

It is often difficult to work out where the major part of the risk for disease comes from. For example, it is well established that living in a city, in general, carries a greater risk of heart disease when compared to living in a rural area. But where are the health hazards associated with living in a city coming from? The environment in the city might be more polluted; however, city living could also be more stressful for some people. A fast-paced lifestyle could lead to poor nutrition or other unhealthy lifestyle habits. People who live in rural areas could feel a stronger sense of community and emotional support.

Despite these misgivings concerning the ability to precisely separate out the risks, sufficient data from around the world points to

environmental influences as real and significant contributing factors
to heart disease.

Passive Smoking

When we think of environmental pollution, naturally we tend to
think of the by-products of the energy industries and motor vehicle exhaust fumes. However, it is also worth mentioning another
environmental pollutant that we might not immediately include
within this category: pollution of the body from secondhand cigarette smoke (passive smoking). Although passive smoking in many
countries might now be less of a problem than it used to be due to
legislation against smoking in public places, it is still a significant risk
for some people.

Large studies have found that passive smoking increases the risk
of coronary heart disease by about 25 percent relative to people not
exposed to the smoke.[53] Unfortunately, these types of studies tend
to publish the results only as relative percentages, rather than absolute percentages. The 25 percent increase in risk is relative to the
baseline risk. For example, if someone has a 10 percent baseline risk
of suffering a heart attack within the next five years, then passive
smoking might increase their risk to 12.5 percent. And if someone
has a baseline risk of 4 percent, passive smoking might increase
their risk of a heart attack to only 5 percent. It's difficult to get a
handle on the real risks for individual population groups without
the absolute percentages.

We can say that, in general, the risks occur after being exposed
to the smoke passively for a duration of about ten years, and on
average, exposure to about twenty cigarettes per day.[3] We also know
that 70–80 percent of the deaths attributable to passive smoking
are caused by heart disease, with less than 5 percent caused by
lung cancer.[54] Therefore, we can postulate that the tissues of the

cardiovascular system are more susceptible than any other part of the body to damage from environmental chemicals and pollutants.

Ambient Air Particles

Pollution in ambient air is defined as anything solid or liquid suspended in the air, including smoke, fumes, soot, and other combustion by-products. It also includes natural particles such as windblown dust, pollen, and spores.

Some of these pollutants are primary particles coming directly out of exhaust stacks and tailpipes, while others are secondary particles such as sulfates and nitrates from condensation of vaporized materials, or from by-products of the oxidation of gases in the atmosphere.[55] Therefore, ambient air can contain a wide range, or mixture, of contaminants from different sources.

Particles are characterized by their aerodynamic properties, measured as their aerodynamic diameter in micrometers (μm). Table 5.2 summarizes the types of particles often present in ambient air and their respective size.

In the mid-1980s, studies of the deposition and clearance of particles in the respiratory system, along with studies of atmospheric physics and chemistry, suggested that smaller particles might be associated with a larger part of the health hazard. Inhalable particles were defined as particulate matter less than 10 μm aerodynamic diameter (PM_{10}). And since the 1990s, evidence has emerged to suggest that even smaller particles, those less than 2.5 μm ($PM_{2.5}$), are able to penetrate into the alveolar gas-exchange regions of the lungs, and that these smaller particles might be particularly hazardous to health.[58]

Modest increases in the level of pollution in the form of $PM_{2.5}$ particles has been associated with an increase in heart disease and heart disease deaths in a number of studies.[56-59] The increased risk is typically around 18–28 percent, but one study did find the risk to be much higher and to be greater in women than in men.[60] Modest increases in the amount of $PM_{2.5}$ have also been linked with changes in heart rate variability (mainly reductions).[61–64]

Problems associated with air pollution are by no means trivial. A World Health Organization (WHO) study that was updated in 2016 stated that more than 80 percent of people living in urban areas that monitor air pollution are exposed to pollution levels that exceed WHO limits.[65] The study included data from 3,000 cities across 103 countries. All regions of the world are affected, although, as we might expect, low-income cities are affected more; 98 percent of cities in low- and middle-income countries, compared to 56 percent of cities in high-income countries, exceed WHO air-quality limits.

The fact that most people in the world breathe air that is considered unsafe is something that should be talked about more. As the WHO states: "As urban air quality declines, the risk of stroke, heart disease, lung cancer, and chronic and acute respiratory diseases, including asthma, increases."

Solar Wind and Geomagnetic Storms

Human biology is, naturally, in tune with the sun in many ways. Metabolic activities are consistent with the range of temperatures on earth influenced by the sun, while the maximum sensitivity of the eye is adjusted to the green wavelengths that are at the peak of the sun's spectral output.[66] Therefore, relatively small changes in the sun's activity could have a significant effect on human health.

A coronal mass ejection (CME) is a burst of solar wind that can disturb the earth's magnetic field when it hits. Some countries can witness the effects through the spectacular aurora borealis (northern lights). The associated increase in geomagnetic energy during a CME has been shown to increase the number of heart attacks

Table 5.2. Constituents of Ambient Air

	Aerodynamic diameter μmol/L		
	ULTRAFINE (0.001−0.1)	PM$_{2.5}$ (0.1−2.5)	PM$_{10}$ (>2.5)
COMPOSITION	Primary combustion products	Aggregates of UFP and vapors; contain most of the sulfates, ammonium compounds, hydro-carbons, elemental carbon, toxic metals	Dust, ground materials, endotoxin, pollen grains, fungal spores, vegetation debris, oxides of Si, Fe, Ca, Al
ORIGIN	Fresh emissions and secondary / photochemical formation	Gas-to-particle conversion, nucleation, and condensation	Suspension in air, sea, spray; grinding, and erosion
SOURCE	Diesel (20−30nm) / Gasoline (20−60nm)	Combustion particles, smog, diesel, gasoline	Windblown soil, agriculture and surface mining, volcanoes, plants
LIFETIME	Minutes to hours	Days	Hours to days
BIOLOGICAL PENETRATION	Alveoli and systemic circulation	Deep lung	Extrathoracic and upper-bronchial regions

Adapted from Bhatnagar, A. Environmental cardiology: studying mechanistic links between pollution and heart disease. *Circ Res.* 2006;99:692–705.

and strokes. Astonishingly, science has known about this since 1922, when a *New York Times* article reported on the work of French doctors who had found that sun spots have an effect on the heart, liver, intestines, and blood vessels.[67] The work was later advanced by Bernhard and Gertraud Düll, a husband and wife research team,[68] and the connection between increased solar activity and increased heart attacks and strokes has now been confirmed in studies done in Russia,[69] Mexico,[70] Cuba,[71] Lithuania,[72] and the United States,[73] among other countries.

In general, these and other studies have found a 10–12 percent increase in the risk of heart attacks on days with increased solar activity. Most of the studies in this area have been secondary prevention research, examining the effect on people who already have some kind of heart problem. It appears that the increased risk only applies to people who have an underlying problem or already have an inappropriately stressed cardiovascular system. Such people are about 10–12 percent more likely, in relative terms, to have a heart attack on days when solar activity is greater. The effects on the heart in this case again seem to be related to heart rate variability. Geomagnetic storms decrease heart rate variability.[73,74]

Although geomagnetic effects are unlikely to be a primary cause of heart disease, the risks are worth mentioning; they provide yet another example illustrating that heart disease is not a simple plumbing problem and that the cardiovascular system (like all the body's systems) is affected by subtle energies that we do not yet fully understand.

CHAPTER SIX

CoQ10 and the
Heart's Energy Factory

The heart gets the energy it needs mainly from tiny energy-producing factories that are contained within the heart muscle itself, called mitochondria (see figure 6.1). Because of the high energy requirements of the heart, the heart contains more mitochondria

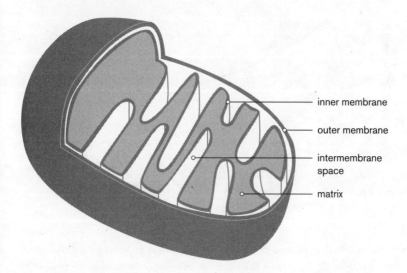

— inner membrane

— outer membrane

— intermembrane space

— matrix

Figure 6.1. Basic structure of mitochondria.

than anywhere else in the body. Each heart muscle cell contains a few thousand mitochondria and these mitochondria account for about 40 percent of the internal space of heart cells.

Mitochondria take the foods we eat, along with oxygen, and convert these into energy via a complex sequence of biochemical actions. Using substances contained in the matrix of the mitochondria, these energy factories convert food into an energy form that the body can use, units of which are called adenosine triphosphate (ATP).

ATP is often described as the correct currency of energy for the body. It provides the energy for just about all biological function, including growth, movement, detoxification, and electrical signaling. Mitochondrial function is an important aspect of heart health; well-functioning mitochondria enable the heart to efficiently pump blood around the body, something that is of obvious importance with regard to heart failure.[1]

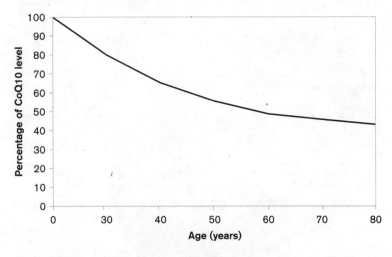

Figure 6.2. Age-related decline in CoQ10 levels in heart tissue. Adapted from Mantle, D. Coenzyme Q10 and cardiovascular disease: an overview. *Br J Cardiol* 2015;22:160.

Conceivably, there are a number of factors that could affect mitochondrial function and, hence, the strength of the heart. Unfortunately, and surprisingly, there has not been a great deal of interest in studying mitochondrial dysfunction in heart failure.[2] The exception to this is the study of coenzyme Q10 (CoQ10), which has implications both for the potential causes of heart disease and for the dangers of statin medications.

CoQ10 is a naturally occurring vitamin-like substance that is a key component of the production of ATP. CoQ10 is involved in the conversion of sugars and fats into this useable form of energy. Therefore, mitochondria are reliant on maintaining adequate amounts of CoQ10 in order to function properly, and in addition to containing more mitochondria than other cells of the body the heart also contains the highest concentrations of CoQ10.

CoQ10 levels within the body decline as we age (see figure 6.2). Even by the age of thirty the availability of CoQ10 has already significantly diminished. Some medical conditions, as well as physical or psychological stress, can also increase the demands for CoQ10. And it is well-known that statin medications block the production of CoQ10 in all cells of the body as discussed earlier.

All things considered, there is good reason to believe that nearly everyone concerned about heart disease is deficient in CoQ10 to some extent because of natural age-related decline in CoQ10 levels, stress-related depletion, a specific health condition, or because of statins.

Supplemental CoQ10

Considerable evidence now exists to confirm the heart health benefits associated with CoQ10 supplementation. Some of the most dramatic results were found in a Swedish study published in 2013 that included 440 people aged seventy to eighty-eight who were split into two groups; one group received a placebo, while the other group received supplemental selenium and CoQ10.[3] After five years, those in the placebo group had a cardiovascular death rate of 12.6 percent, while those in the group who received selenium and CoQ10 had a cardiovascular death rate of 5.9 percent. This dramatic reduction in cardiovascular mortality is considerably greater than any reduction ever seen in a statin clinical trial.

As mentioned previously, in some clinical trials statin medications have been shown to reduce cardiovascular deaths by about 1 percent or 2 percent in absolute terms, but in others the statins did not reduce cardiovascular-related deaths at all.[4,5] In addition, statins have been shown to have even less benefit (in fact, no benefit at all) for the elderly. The Swedish study involving selenium and CoQ10 showed a reduction in cardiovascular deaths of more than 6.5 percent in absolute terms, a reduction in risk that statin supporters can only dream about.

The elderly are even more vulnerable to the adverse effects of statins, particularly because of statin-related depletion of CoQ10. There is also a very strong and well-established connection, which is apparent in the elderly, between low cholesterol levels and increased cancer deaths and deaths from all causes, whereas supplemental CoQ10 could be protective against cancer.[6,7] Whichever way we look at it, CoQ10 supplementation is a much better prospect for the elderly than statins.

The people who were given the selenium and CoQ10 supplements in the Swedish study also performed better than the placebo group in various heart function tests, again confirming the overall benefits associated with the nutrients.

CoQ10 and Selenium

Some CoQ10 is obtained from the diet, but about 75 percent of the body's requirements are made within the body itself, primarily in the liver. The synthesis of CoQ10 requires the presence of a number of amino acids, vitamins, and other nutrients.

There are two different forms of CoQ10, ubiquinone (oxidized form) and ubiquinol (reduced form),[3] both of which are important and each elegantly recycled into the other form within the body with the help of selenium.[8] This helps to explain the benefits seen in the Swedish study; the addition of the selenium probably increased the effectiveness or absorption of the CoQ10.[3]

It is difficult to ascertain what proportion of the benefits seen in the Swedish study could be attributed to the selenium. Low levels of selenium have been associated with an increased risk of heart disease and a shorter life span, while higher levels have been associated with less cancer.[9,10] However, this data is based on observational studies, so the results should be interpreted with some caution.

In fact, selenium supplementation has been shown to exhibit a U-shaped curve; people with low levels of selenium receive benefit, but people with adequate or high levels can actually experience adverse effects from additional selenium.[11]

Swedish people are known to have low levels of selenium,[11,12] so in this case, at least part of the benefits seen in the study were likely to be attributable to the selenium. However, in terms of a universal therapy, widespread selenium supplementation could be appropriate for Swedes but not necessarily for other populations.

CoQ10 and Heart Failure

Congestive heart failure is the inability of the heart to adequately circulate blood around the body. In the 1970s, Per Langsjoen, Karl Folkers, and Gian Paolo Littarru undertook pioneering studies on CoQ10 and heart failure. They found that blood and cardiac tissue levels of CoQ10 were lower in people with heart failure. Later, Per

Langsjoen, Per's son Peter Langsjoen, and Karl Folkers completed the first clinical study in this area, which included 144 patients with heart failure who were followed for six years.[13] The results were extremely encouraging, showing improvement in 85 percent of patients.

Dr. Peter Langsjoen has continued to work with CoQ10 for many years in his cardiology practice in Tyler, Texas, and has published a number of articles on the use of CoQ10 in cardiovascular disease.[14,15] Overall, there is now an extensive and growing body of evidence showing the effectiveness of CoQ10 in treating heart failure.[16–19]

Some evidence suggests that CoQ10 supplementation needs to be taken over a certain period of time in order to achieve significant cardiovascular benefits. A study published in the *Journal of the American College of Cardiology* in 2014 found no significant improvements in markers for heart function associated with CoQ10 after sixteen weeks of treatment, but after two years the benefits were dramatic.[20] The study included 420 patients with severe heart failure, split into two groups receiving either CoQ10 or placebo, respectively, in addition to the standard medications that are used for this condition. Overall, those people given the CoQ10 had almost half the number of major adverse cardiac events (MACE) and almost half the number of cardiovascular related deaths and deaths from all causes (see table 6.1).

The category of MACE was the primary focus of the study, so it is worth taking a slightly more detailed look at it. MACE was defined to include heart attack deaths, heart failure deaths, sudden cardiac deaths, and hospital admissions for worsening heart failure. One of the most striking findings was the difference in heart failure deaths. In the placebo group, 10 people died of heart failure, whereas 1 person died of heart failure in the CoQ10 group. There were also half the number of hospital admissions due to heart failure in the CoQ10 group.

Table 6.1. Summary of the Results of a Study Investigating the Use of CoQ10 in Patients with Severe Heart Failure (Follow-up for Two Years)[22]

	Placebo group (%)	CoQ10 group (%)
Major adverse cardiac events (MACE)	26	15
Cardiovascular-related deaths	16	9
Deaths from all causes	18	10

Source: Alberts B, Johnson A, Lewis J, et al. *Molecular biology of the cell. 4th edition.* New York: Garland Science; 2002.

Supporters of the mass prescription of statin medications in the United Kingdom have often said that statins save 10,000 lives each year in England.[21] This number is extrapolated from clinical trials and is based on around 7 million people taking statins. We could do a similar extrapolation based on the CoQ10 study mentioned above. Using the United States as an example, where there are an estimated 5.7 million people with heart failure, if all of those people were given supplemental CoQ10, extrapolating from the above study, more than 60,000 lives would be saved each year from heart failure alone, at least six times more lives saved than with statins, and with fewer people treated (5.7 million people compared with 7 million). Unlike statins, which have a long list of common adverse effects, the only side effects associated with CoQ10 are likely to be improvements in other areas of health.

Obviously, much larger studies would need to be done to confirm the benefits of the use of CoQ10 on this scale; however, this comparison is valid in that it helps to put the suggested benefits of statins into perspective, and it also shows that incredibly promising alternative treatments are currently being neglected.

Other Heart Benefits

The inside walls of the blood vessels are lined with endothelial cells. These cells perform a number of important functions, including reacting to changes in shear stress and releasing nitric oxide to allow the vessel to dilate in order to increase blood flow.[22] Studies investigating CoQ10 supplementation and endothelial function have been somewhat inconsistent. In addition, some studies have involved a very small number of people and were conducted over a very short duration. However, a meta-analysis of these studies published in the journal *Atherosclerosis* in 2012 found that endothelial function of the arteries was significantly improved with CoQ10 supplementation, in patients both with and without existing cardiovascular disease.[23]

The positive effect on the function of the endothelium, inducing vasodilation, has the additional benefit of lowering blood pressure. A number of studies have shown that CoQ10 supplementation can be an effective agent for lowering blood pressure in hypertensive patients.[24-26] And, again, this positive effect comes without the side effects normally experienced with the medications that are typically used for lowering blood pressure.

CoQ10 as an Antioxidant

Antioxidants are used by the body to prevent cellular damage due to free radicals, which are atoms that have an unbalanced number of electrons. Free radicals are unstable and try to "steal" the nearest electron in order to become balanced. But this action creates a new free radical and a cascade of reactions that can disrupt the cell. Antioxidants "donate" an electron without becoming a free radical themselves, putting a stop to the free radicals.

A balance between free radicals and antioxidants is necessary for proper physiological function. A condition known as oxidative stress results if the body cannot cope with free radicals; this condition can have serious implications for health and is implicated in a number of degenerative diseases.[27]

CoQ10 is an important antioxidant. It is a frontline antioxidant in that the body tends to use CoQ10 first, before using other antioxidants.

How Much and Which Form?

CoQ10 supplements are available in both the ubiquinone and ubiquinol forms. The ubiquinone form is generally more easily available in stores and is less expensive than ubiquinol. Most of the clinical trials completed on CoQ10 have used the ubiquinone form. In theory, if ubiquinone is consumed, the body can convert this into ubiquinol, but some people (for example, the elderly and those with chronic medical conditions) might not be able to efficiently convert ubiquinone into ubiquinol, and therefore they need to take the ubiquinol form in order to experience the full benefits.

Patients with severe heart failure might not be able to absorb ubiquinone because of intestinal edema. Dr. Peter Langsjoen, along with his wife, Alena, conducted the first clinical trial using ubiquinol with critically ill heart failure patients.[15] These patients previously only had very limited clinical improvement with ubiquinone supplementation, but ubiquinol resulted in a significant increase in blood levels and a corresponding dramatic improvement in symptoms and heart function.

As with all nutrients, each person has unique requirements. Ideally, CoQ10 supplementation should be taken in conjunction with blood tests to monitor levels and tailor the therapy accordingly. This approach was taken by Dr. Langsjoen, with the use of an onsite laboratory for measuring CoQ10 levels. In general, the studies mentioned in this chapter have used a dosage of between 120 and 600 mg per day. Since not all of the CoQ10 can be absorbed in one go, it is better to spread the dose out into two or three smaller doses taken throughout the day to maximize the absorption. CoQ10 is also best taken with food containing fat or oil.

There are no known serious adverse effects of CoQ10 supplementation and no known toxic effects. CoQ10 cannot be overdosed, and as much as 900 mg per day is well tolerated in adults.[3] Two studies investigating the use of CoQ10 in Parkinson's and Alzheimer's disease used a dose of 3,000 mg per day without any adverse effects.[28,29]

Although health authorities have for the last fifty years been pushing the idea that animal fats are unhealthy, the best food sources of CoQ10 are animal proteins. The highest concentrations of CoQ10 are found in organ meats such as beef, chicken, and pork hearts and liver, though these foods have become less palatable for many people as food trends have changed over time. Beef and pork in general are also good sources of CoQ10. So are sardines, mackerel, and herrings. Plant-based foods generally contain less CoQ10, but notable sources include peanuts, sesame seeds, walnuts, pistachio nuts, hazelnuts, spinach, broccoli, avocado, and cauliflower.

It is astonishing that the ability of the heart to generate energy is not even remotely considered by health authorities when assessing a person's risk for heart disease. Mitochondrial health and CoQ10 levels are obviously important determining factors in a range of different heart conditions, yet this is currently not considered by health authorities or the cardiovascular risk calculators. Instead, these authorities have sanctioned expensive and toxic medications for hundreds of millions of people worldwide.

CHAPTER SEVEN

Nutrition for the Heart

There are a seemingly infinite number of ways that our nutritional status can affect our heart health, for good or ill. Some nutritional factors have been established and reported on for many years, while the effects of other nutritional factors are less clear and more debatable. Many additional nutritional factors doubtlessly remain to be discovered. This chapter discusses the nutritional aspects that we already know are important for the prevention of heart disease, as well as the nutritional interventions that have been shown to be more effective than statin medications.

Macronutrients

It is logical to first look at the importance of macronutrients, substances of which we eat relatively large amounts, such as proteins, fats, and carbohydrates. However, we will mostly focus on the latter two, as they have been more extensively studied in relation to cardiovascular risk than protein has.

We all know the advice: We should avoid eating too much fat, particularly saturated fat. The idea is that when we eat too much fat we get fat. However, dietary trials have contradicted this idea, consistently finding that increasing the fat content of the diet actually results in more weight loss.[1-6]

In addition, for decades it has been suggested that eating fat will increase the amount of fats in the blood and contribute to a clogging of the arteries. Fats in the bloodstream are called triglycerides. Having high levels of triglycerides is a bad sign; this is a common feature of diabetes and people with diabetes are up to five times more likely to have heart disease than are people who don't have diabetes. But high triglyceride levels are not caused by a high-fat diet.

At least eleven dietary trials found that a low-fat diet, not a high-fat diet, caused levels of triglycerides to increase,[1,4-13] and no studies have found that increased dietary fat increases triglyceride levels. Initially, this might seem to be counterintuitive; however, it makes sense when we consider how the body actually works.

A low-fat diet by definition includes more carbohydrates. Once eaten and absorbed into the body, carbohydrates become glucose in the bloodstream. If we eat a lot of carbohydrates, blood glucose levels can become too high, prompting the body to prioritize rectifying this situation, because high blood glucose levels cause circulatory problems and damage to the inside walls of blood vessels. Blood glucose triggers the release of the hormone insulin, which lowers blood glucose levels and enables the body's cells to use the glucose. But if there is too much glucose, the excess glucose is converted into fat in the bloodstream (triglycerides). This explains why low-fat/high-carbohydrate diets increase blood triglyceride levels, as well as why, possibly alongside other mechanisms, high blood glucose levels have been established as an independent risk factor for heart disease, not just for people with diabetes but for everyone. The risk increases as blood glucose levels increase, starting at about a 10 percent increased risk up to a 30 percent increased risk as blood glucose levels rise, after which point we reach the diabetic threshold whereby the cardiovascular risks associated with high blood glucose rapidly increase even further.[14–25] The cardiovascular risk score used by doctors (which is supposed to accurately predict each person's individual risk for a cardiovascular problem) includes diabetes as a risk factor but docs not take into account blood glucose levels below the diabetic threshold.

In addition to being told to eat a low-fat diet, we are also told that a low level of so-called good cholesterol (HDLs) is a risk factor for heart disease (a person's HDL level is included in current cardiovascular risk calculators). But low-fat diets have repeatedly been shown to lower HDL levels.[1,4,5,7,8,10,13,26–28] The belief that a higher HDL level is protective is not consistent with the belief that a low-fat diet is healthy; they are mutually exclusive and an example of dietary doublethink, revealing the absurd nature of the current guidelines and the current model of heart disease prevention.

Fish and Essential Fatty Acids

The general nutritional perception is that eating fish is good for the heart, with Japan sometimes referred to as an example in support of this idea, because its cuisine is known to feature large amounts of fish and its citizens have an extremely low rate of heart disease. However, the Japanese diet for the most part stresses fresh and flavorsome ingredients of all kinds, including beef, pork, and chicken, as well as health-promoting fermented foods such as pickles, miso soup, and natto. Therefore it is difficult to determine which parts of the Japanese diet are most cardio-protective. The Japanese also consume a fair amount of white rice, which clouds the picture further when trying to analyze their diet.

Similarly, the Mediterranean diet is sometimes discussed in connection with the benefits of eating fish. But the Mediterranean diet is highly variable. Its high nutrient content and health-promoting benefits can

be attributed to a number of different dietary elements, including fresh
vegetables, which are often consumed in relatively large quantities.

In addition, there are populations of people who do not consume
very much fish but also have a low rate of heart disease: for example,
the people living in the mountain village of Anogia on the island of
Crete (as featured in *Statin Nation II*).

The Nurses Health Study (an observational study that included
around 85,000 women) found that fish consumption was associated
with a reduction in sudden deaths; the number of heart attacks were
not lower in women who consumed more fish, but the overall heart
disease death rate was lower.[29,30] Yet again, we cannot be sure the
extent to which other factors played a role.

The question here is not about whether or not fish consumption
is, in general, healthy, which it is, but rather, whether or not fish
offers any extra cardio-protectiveness over and above alternative
foods such as meat or poultry. It is difficult to say that it does.

Historically, fish has been considered healthier for the heart than
beef, pork, and chicken because it contains less saturated fat. We
now know that saturated fat does not cause heart disease. Certain
types of fish are also said to be good for the heart because of the
essential fatty acids they contain. Essential fatty acids (EFAs) are
fats that the body cannot make by itself and they therefore must be
obtained from the diet on a regular basis. Whether or not EFAs are
cardio-protective can be considered separately from the discussion
about fish consumption because other foods also contain EFAs.

Two EFAs, omega-3 and omega-6, have received a great deal
of attention in the media. Just how much omega-3 and omega-6
the human body needs is still unclear; however, we do know that
consuming more of one than the other is detrimental to health.
Omega-3 and omega-6 have opposing properties. Omega-3 reduces
inflammation and helps blood to flow more easily through the

blood vessels and arteries. This is exactly what is needed in order to help prevent heart disease. However, the consumption of too much omega-3 will make it difficult for the body to produce blood clots in the event of any damage to the tissues, leading to excessive bleeding. This is where omega-6 comes in, which helps blood coagulate in order to stop bleeding at the site of an injury. Clearly, the body requires a balance of omega-3 and omega-6.

It is generally agreed that most people in industrialized countries consume too much omega-6. This is because omega-6 is found in relatively large quantities in vegetable oils (such as sunflower oil) and in grain-based foods such as cereals, bread, and pasta, the consumption of which has increased during the last few decades. Omega-3 is primarily obtained from oily fish, but some omega-3 is also found in grass-fed beef.

Overconsumption of omega-6 compared to omega-3 is associated with an increased risk for heart disease and other degenerative conditions.[31] This would seem to make the case for supplementing one's diet with omega-3. Indeed, the GISSI study[32] found a benefit associated with supplementing with omega-3 for people who had already suffered a heart attack. The GISSI study followed more than 11,000 people for three and a half years, reporting on a range of cardiovascular events. For example, under the classification of coronary heart disease deaths and nonfatal heart attacks, 9.2 percent of the people not given the omega-3 supplementation suffered these events, versus 6.9 percent of people given omega-3 (the omega-3 group were given 1 gram of omega-3 per day).

The mechanisms by which omega-3 could reduce the risk for further heart problems are still being debated. Risk reduction could be due to the anticoagulation properties of omega-3, as discussed above.

The benefits of omega-3 supplementation shown in the GISSI study are at least as good as, if not better than, the results that have been seen in clinical trials done on statins in secondary prevention, where we have typically seen a general cardiovascular risk reduction of about 2 percent for people who have already had a heart attack.[33] However, other studies have thus far failed to find any benefit associated with omega-3 supplementation.[34]

Too much omega-3 could also pose a problem, but any risks associated with omega-3 supplementation are likely to be far less severe than the adverse effects associated with statins. Therefore, on balance, omega-3 supplementation can be considered as part of an overall nutritional protocol that replaces statins.

Fruits and Vegetables

As we've discussed, too many carbohydrates in the diet have the effect of raising blood glucose levels and increasing the risk of heart disease. However, it is mostly carbohydrates in the form of grain-based foods (such as bread, pasta, and rice) and sugars that have this effect. Vegetables do not cause large fluctuations in blood glucose. Some starchy vegetables (such as potatoes) can affect blood glucose to some extent, but in general, vegetables are the best carbohydrates for stabilizing blood glucose levels.

Increased vegetable consumption has consistently been linked with reduced risk of heart disease, both within populations and when vegetable consumption is compared across different countries.[35,36] These findings could just be an association, with other factors playing more important roles; however, there are many biologically plausible reasons why vegetables are good for the heart. Aside from the fact that they help us to maintain stable blood glucose levels, vegetables also contain some important nutrients for the heart and blood vessels, vitamin C in particular. We need to eat fruits and vegetables every day in order to get enough vitamin C into our bodies, which is important for the integrity of the inside wall of the arteries, and which we will discuss in more detail later in this chapter. Some vegetables also contain high amounts of magnesium, which is extremely important for optimal heart function and normalizing blood pressure, as we will also see.

There is evidence that cruciferous vegetables are particularly good for the heart.[37] These include arugula, broccoli, bok choy, Brussels sprouts, cabbage, collards, cauliflower, horseradish, kale, kohlrabi, mustard greens, radishes, rutabaga, turnips (and their greens), wasabi, and watercress.

As an aside to the discussion of vegetables, just to set the record straight: meat, poultry, seafood, and eggs are also important sources of essential nutrients. These foods, in general, provide the best sources for vitamins A, D, B_1, B_2, B_3, B_6, B_{12}, pantothenic acid, biotin, coenzyme Q10, and saturated fatty acids.[38] We can see that animal- and plant-based foods complement each other to provide all of the nutrients humans need for good health.

As with all things, different people react in different ways to fruits. Fruits are generally healthy, and increased fruit consumption is also linked with a reduced risk of heart disease.[35,36] However, many health practitioners feel that eating too much fruit can bring blood glucose levels out of balance, at least for some people. Fruit contains a lot of sugar, and at a certain level of fruit consumption, depending on the individual, the high sugar intake from the fruit can increase blood glucose levels and counter fruits' otherwise health-promoting qualities.

As a general guide, feeling hungry soon after eating fruit is a good indication that one's metabolism is sensitive to the sugars in fruit, and therefore fruit intake should be limited. The real danger, however, is associated with fruit juice. A piece of fruit contains fiber that helps slow down the absorption of the sugar. Juicing removes the fiber, which means the body gets a massive sugar hit in just a few gulps.

Homocysteine and B Vitamins

Homocysteine is a naturally occurring substance in the blood, high levels of which have been linked in a number of studies with an increased risk of heart disease. It was established some time ago that taking supplemental folic acid, vitamin B_6, and vitamin B_{12} lowers homocysteine levels.[39] Understandably, these findings led to a fair amount of excitement and anticipation, since the results suggested simply adding these supplements to the diet could significantly reduce heart disease risk.

A number of clinical trials have now been conducted whereby people with existing heart disease have been given folic acid, vitamin B_6, and vitamin B_{12} supplements. In each case homocysteine levels have been lowered, but unfortunately, none of the studies have shown any actual direct cardiovascular benefit.

The Norwegian Vitamin Trial (NORVIT), for example, included 3,749 men and women who had suffered a heart attack within seven days prior to the start of the trial.[40] Participants were split into four groups: a vitamin B_6 group; a folic acid and vitamin B_{12} group; a folic acid, vitamin B_{12}, and vitamin B_6 group; and a placebo group. After about forty months, the researchers looked at the data and found that although homocysteine levels had been reduced significantly, there was no evidence of this translating into any actual cardiovascular benefit.

The Heart Outcomes Prevention Evaluation (HOPE-2) trial, which included 5,522 patients with vascular disease or diabetes, found similar results: a reduction in homocysteine but no reduction in heart attacks, although this trial also saw a reduction in the number of nonfatal strokes in the group who took folic acid, vitamin B_6, and vitamin B_{12}.[41]

Another trial included 5,442 female health professionals in the United States who had either a history of cardiovascular disease or three or more heart disease risk factors. Participants were given folic acid, vitamin B_6, and vitamin B_{12}, or a placebo, for seven years. Again, homocysteine levels were reduced, but this did not translate into heart health benefits.[42]

For the most part, participants in these trials have, at the same time as taking the supplements, been taking a range of cardiovascular medications. Therefore the possibility of some kind of interaction between the medications and the supplements could exist. But overall, homocysteine looks like it could be another example of what happens when we focus on suggested individual risk factors. Homocysteine is certainly involved in the processes associated with heart disease, but it remains to be seen if it can be an effective target for treatment. It could simply be associated with other risk factors that as yet remain unknown.

L-Arginine

L-arginine is an amino acid that converts into nitric oxide. Nitric oxide is an extremely important substance; it dilates the blood vessels and is therefore critical for circulation. Because of this, L-arginine has become a popular nutritional supplement, especially for people with high blood pressure.

However, when I interviewed Professor Sherif Sultan, one of the world's leading vascular and endovascular surgeons, for *Statin Nation II*, he explained that L-arginine supplementation has been shown to cause a number of adverse effects. L-arginine can cause some types of cancer to spread, for example. Some forms of irregular heartbeat can also be made worse by L-arginine, and L-arginine can actually cause blood pressure to become dangerously low for some people.

A study published in the *Journal of the American Medical Association* in 2006 looked at the effect of giving L-arginine to patients after they had suffered a heart attack. It found that L-arginine, surprisingly, did not improve vascular stiffness measurements. In fact, six patients in the L-arginine group died during the six-month trial compared with no deaths in the placebo group. The researchers understandably concluded that "L-Arginine should not be recommended following acute myocardial infarction."[43]

Vitamin C

Vitamin C (ascorbic acid) can be made internally by most animals, using glucose as the raw material. Glucose is converted into ascorbic acid in the liver via a step-by-step sequence of biochemical actions, the last of which requires the enzyme L-gulonogammalactone oxidase (GLO).

As a result of genetic mutations, humans (along with a few other animals, such as some higher primates, guinea pigs, and an Indian fruit-eating bat) can no longer produce GLO and hence cannot internally make vitamin C. Humans must therefore obtain adequate amounts of vitamin C through their diet. Failure to do so results in scurvy.

The theory behind our inability to produce vitamin C is that the gene for producing the GLO enzyme was lost in a primate ancestor some 50 million years ago, which has led to some researchers referring to scurvy as a genetic disorder.[44]

Scurvy was mentioned by Hippocrates,[44,45] and ancient Egyptians had several hieroglyphs to describe the disease.[45-47] Over the course of history, the cure for scurvy has in various forms been discovered, forgotten, and rediscovered again several times. Of particular interest is the work of James Lind, a Scottish physician who, during the eighteenth century, was a pioneer of naval hygiene. Lind discovered, by conducting the world's first-ever clinical trial, that giving citrus fruits to sailors prevented scurvy. Lind's prospective controlled experiment, which he carried out in 1747, involved comparing the relative benefits of six treatments for scurvy used at the time.[48] The two sailors who were given citrus fruits exhibited an almost complete remission within just a few days. We now know that these dramatic results were due to the vitamin C content of the fruits (see tables 7.1 and 7.2, pages 114 and 115, for the vitamin C content of various fruits and vegetables).

James Lind's work is of note because it was the first controlled experiment. However, the cure for scurvy was actually discovered forty years earlier by Ebbot Michell. In her handwritten book dated 1707, Michell details a recipe for curing scurvy, which involves mixing the extracts of various medicinal plants (some of them rich in vitamin C) with orange juice.[49] The book was discovered in 2009 in a house in Gloucestershire, England. Ebbot Michell is not yet mentioned in medical historical texts, but one hopes this will be corrected and Michell's contribution will be acknowledged in future texts. The Admiralty did not adopt the recommendations of Michell or Lund until 1795. During the decades of delay, thousands of sailors died prematurely of scurvy.

Vitamin C also has an important role to play in the prevention of heart disease. To understand this, we must discuss vitamin C's role in the production of collagen.

Collagen

Collagen is the major fibrous protein that basically keeps our bodies together, and is the most abundant protein in the animal kingdom. It is a major part of the connective tissue and provides the structural components outside the cells of the body. It is also found inside certain cells; collagen has high tensile strength and composes the main part of ligaments, tendons, cartilage, bones, teeth, and other parts of the body. Collagen strengthens blood vessels and helps tissues to withstand stretching.

There are at least sixteen types of collagen, but 80–90 percent of the collagen in the body is type I, II, or III.[50] Figure 7.1 depicts a magnified image of collagen fibers. Scurvy is basically tissue breakdown caused by not having the ability to make enough collagen. Early symptoms of scurvy include muscle and joint pain, tiredness, generally not feeling well or constantly feeling miserable, and the appearance of red dots on the skin. If adequate amounts of vitamin C are not consumed to correct this, then further symptoms appear, such as swelling and bleeding of the gums, more severe joint pain, shortness of breath, and a significantly impaired ability to heal wounds.

The inside walls of our blood vessels are lined with endothelial cells. These cells perform a number of important functions, including reacting to changes in shear stress and releasing nitric oxide to allow the vessel to dilate in order to increase blood flow.[51] Collagen is essential for the integrity of these cells (the endothelium). Collagen type I also influences the shape of the endothelial cells.[52] If the

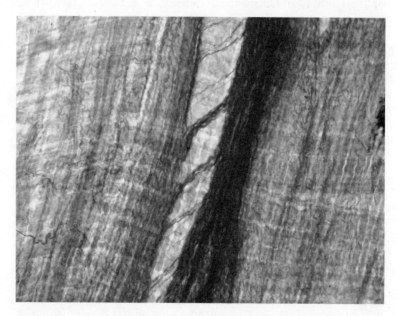

Figure 7.1. Magnified image of collagen fibers perfectly arranged in two directions. Image courtesy of Ganimedes/Wikimedia Commons.

body cannot produce enough collagen, it could become difficult to maintain the integrity of the inside wall of the blood vessels. This is particularly important for the coronary arteries, which supply blood and oxygen to the heart. The coronary arteries are connected to the side of the heart, which is continuously beating and contracting, causing the coronary arteries to be continuously squeezed and bent. Sufficient collagen is needed in order to keep the integrity of the endothelium inside the coronary arteries, and to repair any damage.

Locations where arteries bifurcate (split into two branches) are also under greater biomechanical stress, because they are places where the blood becomes more turbulent. And these locations, in particular, require sufficient collagen to maintain the integrity of the endothelium.

The coronary arteries and artery bifurcations (the areas that are more susceptible to structural damage) are also the places where atherosclerosis (the buildup of arterial plaque) often occurs.

In short, if there is insufficient vitamin C available to make enough collagen at locations within the artery where high biomechanical stress exists, then damage to the wall of the artery can occur or existing damage cannot be repaired, and blood clots and plaques can form. Heart disease, from this point of view, is effectively a pre-scurvy condition, or a subclinical form of scurvy affecting the arteries.

The theory of coronary heart disease as primarily due to insufficient vitamin C has been championed by Linus Pauling, the double Nobel Laureate, and by Dr. Matthias Rath, who worked with Dr. Pauling. However, another researcher, Irwin Stone, deserves more credit than he has been given to date.

Irwin Stone was an American biochemist and chemical engineer who took a great deal of interest in vitamin C. Stone was responsible for getting Linus Pauling interested in vitamin C when he met him in 1966; Pauling found Stone to be extremely well-informed and convincing.[53] At that time, Stone had already written several papers about vitamin C.

In 1972, Dr. Stone published his classic book *The Healing Factor: Vitamin C Against Disease*,[54] which included a foreword by Linus Pauling and another Nobel Laureate, Albert Szent-Gyorgyi (Szent-Gyorgyi first isolated vitamin C).

There are many parts of Irwin Stone's book that will be of interest to anyone studying nutrition and health, and it is considered an important text on orthomolecular medicine, the application of the right amounts of natural substances to maintain good health. But there is one aspect in particular that is highly relevant to our discussion; it raises some questions that have yet to be answered with regard to the recommended daily amount of vitamin C.

Irwin Stone suggested that the daily amount of vitamin C recommended by health authorities was inadequate. In *The Healing Factor*[54] he states:

> The recommended daily allowance for an adult human for ascorbic acid is 60 milligrams per day (about one milligram per kilogram of body weight). From the Committee on Animal Nutrition's "Nutrient Requirements of Laboratory Animals" (1962) we find some startling figures. The recommended diet for the monkey—our closest mammalian relative—is 55 milligrams of ascorbic acid per kilogram of body weight or 3,830 milligrams of ascorbic acid per day for the average adult human. The daily amount suggested as adequate for the guinea pig varies depending upon which of two diets is selected and ranges from 42 to 167 milligrams per kilogram of body weight (based on a 300-gram guinea pig). This amounts to 2,920 milligrams to 11,650 milligrams per day for the average adult human.

Since Stone's book was published, the recommended daily amount of vitamin C for the United States has increased slightly to 75–120 mg per day for adults.[55,56] In the United Kingdom, the recommended daily amount is 40 mg per day.[57] This has led Linus Pauling and other eminent researchers to suggest that these recommended intake levels are based only on an adequate amount to stay alive and prevent symptoms of scurvy, and that humans require larger amounts of vitamin C daily than the guidelines suggest in order to achieve good health.

In general, Dr. Pauling and others suggest that an intake of several grams per day of vitamin C, rather than 60 mg per day, would be more appropriate for humans.[54] And this is where things start to become a bit trickier.

It is impossible to consume several grams of vitamin C per day by eating normal foods (see tables 7.1 and 7.2). In order to do so, we would need to consume something like twelve full cups of raw peppers per day, or more than fifty oranges. Therefore, the only way to achieve the intake suggested by Dr. Pauling and others is through nutritional supplementation.

Dr. Pauling and Dr. Matthias Rath also went on to further develop their theory by incorporating lipoprotein(a). Lipoprotein(a), or Lp(a), is a combination of the adhesive protein apo(a) with a low-density lipoprotein (LDL) particle. Some epidemiological studies have linked a high level of Lp(a) with an increased risk of cardiovascular disease. Levels of Lp(a) are genetically determined and are not thought to be generally affected by diet.[58] However, some doctors have anecdotally reported a reduction in Lp(a) levels after nutrition and lifestyle changes.

Pauling and Rath believe that Lp(a) is increased as a compensatory mechanism because of the genetic limitations causing a deficiency in vitamin C in humans. Pauling and Rath observed that Lp(a) is mainly only increased in animals that cannot make their own vitamin C.[59]

Table 7.1. Vitamin C in Servings of Vegetables, from Most to Least

Vegetable	Serving	Vitamin C (in mg)
Red and Green peppers, cooked	½ cup	121–132
Red and yellow peppers, raw	½ cup	101–144
Green peppers, raw	½ cup	63
Broccoli, cooked	½ cup	54
Red cabbage, raw	1 cup	54
Kohlrabi, cooked	½ cup	47
Broccoli, raw	½ cup	42
Snow peas, cooked	½ cup	41
Brussels sprouts, cooked	4 sprouts	38–52
Cabbage, cooked	½ cup	30
Kale, cooked	½ cup	28
Cauliflower, raw or cooked	½ cup	26–29
Rapini, cooked	½ cup	24
Bok choy, cooked	½ cup	23
Potato (with skin), cooked	1 medium	22
Sweet potato (with skin), cooked	1 medium	22
Asparagus (from frozen), cooked	6 spears	22
Turnip greens, cooked	½ cup	21
Snow peas, raw	½ cup	20
Collard greens, cooked	½ cup	18
Tomato, raw	1 medium	18
Tomato sauce, canned	½ cup	15

And they hypothesized that Lp(a) is deposited in the artery wall as a substitute for collagen (insufficient collagen being a result of a lack of vitamin C). They presented their theory in a paper titled "A Unified Theory of Human Cardiovascular Disease Leading the Way to

Table 7.2. Vitamin C in Servings of Fruit, from Most to Least

Fruit	Serving	Vitamin C (in mg)
Guava	1 fruit	206
Papaya	½ fruit	94
Kiwi	1 large	84
Orange	1 medium	59–83
Lychee	10 fruits	69
Strawberry	½ cup	52
Pineapple	½ cup	39–49
Grapefruit	½ fruit	38–47
Clementine	1 fruit	36
Cantaloupe	½ cup	31
Mango	½ fruit	29
Avocado	½ fruit	26
Soursop	½ cup	25
Tangerine/mandarin orange	1 medium	22
Balsam pear/bitter melon	½ cup	22
Persimmon	½ cup	17
Berries, general	½ cup	14–17

the Abolition of This Disease as a Cause for Human Mortality."[60,61] This paper, and the theory it presented, are compelling to say the least. The suggestion that vitamin C deficiency is the root cause of all cardiovascular disease was presented very coherently. However, there are a number of important questions that remain unanswered.

Accepting that vitamin C is the main factor in heart disease suggests that many other important factors are less important or irrelevant. Additional intake of vitamin C could provide protection from the effects of some of the other causes of heart disease. For example, vitamin C can help the body repair itself when it is under stress or when other factors are present that might otherwise cause damage to the endothelium. But overall, heart disease involves the complex interaction of many factors rather than just one "unified theory."

Pauling and Rath are not the first talented researchers to become enthralled with their discoveries to the neglect of other important factors. The incorporation of Lp(a) takes us back to the oversimplified risk factor–based approach, with all of its shortcomings. Is the "risk factor" genuinely involved or just a marker for something else?

Based on the unified theory, Pauling and Rath developed a nutritional protocol. The protocol involves supplementing one's diet with large amounts of vitamin C and the amino acid lysine. They suggest that lysine, in sufficient quantities, can prevent Lp(a) from accumulating in the artery wall.

It is important to keep in mind that no clinical trial has specifically tested the effectiveness of the Pauling/Rath protocol for preventing or reversing heart disease. To be fair, it is difficult to test a specific nutritional protocol because there is not a financial incentive for the pharmaceutical companies, who conduct about 85 percent of clinical trials, to do this kind of trial. So, unfortunately, it is unlikely that the Pauling/Rath protocol will be tested in a clinical trial anytime soon.

Although there are not yet any published trials involving the Pauling/Rath protocol exactly, there is some evidence that supplemental vitamin C could reduce the risk of heart disease.

In 2004, *The American Journal of Clinical Nutrition* published an analysis of nine studies that included information on intakes of vitamin E, carotenoids, and vitamin C. The most significant finding was that people who took 700 mg or more of supplemental vitamin C suffered 25 percent fewer heart attacks.[62]

Some people might speculate that if the dose of vitamin C was higher, and closer to what Pauling and Rath recommend, then the reduction in risk might be greater. Of course, we cannot know the effect without testing it; however, supplemental vitamin C at a higher dosage has been shown to provide some encouraging results for people with type 2 diabetes.[63]

In one study, researchers split participants into two groups; one group received 500 mg per day while the other received 1,000 mg per day, for six weeks. Both groups experienced a lowering of blood glucose levels, but the reduction in blood glucose was considerably greater in the 1,000 mg vitamin C group, which also experienced a significant reduction in insulin levels.

Vitamin C is almost always referred to as ascorbic acid, which it is, but vitamin C from whole foods comes in the form of ascorbic acid with bioflavonoids and other biological compounds. Ascorbic acid alone is an isolate, and there is ongoing debate about the merits of using isolates of nutrients.

Most vitamin C supplements are ascorbic acid isolates, synthetically derived in a laboratory. However, an increasing range of vitamin C products are now available that are derived from whole foods, and an increasing number of health practitioners hold the view that these whole food–based supplements are more beneficial. In general, the required dosage of a whole food–based supplement is usually considerably less than that of an isolate because the whole food supplements are thought to be better absorbed.

In summary, supplemental vitamin C at a dosage of 1 gram or more per day could be seriously considered for people with a diagnosed heart problem or type 2 diabetes. These people could also consider the whole food–based supplemental form of vitamin C at a potentially lower dosage.

The most appropriate choice for people who consider themselves to be at high risk (but without a diagnosed heart problem) would probably also be a whole food–based vitamin C supplement. This would also be a good option for people with a chronic illness of any other kind, people with a high-stress lifestyle, and people going through a particularly stressful event.

Vitamin C is generally considered not to be toxic at high levels; however, we might not yet understand all of its synergistic or antagonistic relationships with other nutrients. We should also always keep in mind the concept of biochemical individuality, as described by Dr. Roger Williams,[64] which suggests that megadoses of a nutrient might be required by some people, but not all people. For these reasons it might be prudent to reserve longer-term higher dosage of vitamin C of more than 1 gram per day for those with a diagnosed medical condition, where the risk of any negative effects is likely to be offset by the potential benefits. Even nutritional supplements have risks, although fewer than the risks associated with cholesterol-lowering medications such as statins, which are toxic for everyone, even at the lowest dose.

This information about vitamin C, at the very least, serves as a reminder of the importance of regularly consuming foods containing vitamin C. Vegetables and fruits are the best sources of vitamin C. However, as stated above, obtaining vitamin C in the form of fruit juice is not a good idea because of its high sugar content and because it involves a rapid release of sugar. This fact is even more relevant here because a high sugar intake can impair the absorption of vitamin C. Although Ebbot Michell included orange juice in her remedy for scurvy, we can assume that the sailors she was dosing were consuming considerably less sugar than the average person does today, so this aspect of her remedy could arguably have been less of a concern at that time. Meat, dairy products, and grains do not contain vitamin C, or only in tiny amounts.

The information contained within this chapter refers to vitamin C specifically for the prevention of heart disease. Vitamin C supplementation at a higher dosage could also be applicable to the treatment of other health conditions that are beyond the scope of this book.

Magnesium

Magnesium is one of the most important factors where nutrition and heart health are concerned, but, unfortunately, magnesium deficiency is currently overlooked by most doctors and cardiologists. Magnesium is the eleventh most abundant element in the human body; though it accounts for less than 0.1 percent of the body's mass, it is essential for hundreds of life-sustaining biochemical processes.

Around half of the magnesium in the body is found in the bones; most of the remaining half is found in the tissues and organs, while about 1 percent of the body's magnesium is in the blood.[65-67] Because magnesium is involved in too many biological processes to describe in one book, this section will focus on the biological functions specifically related to heart disease.

Cellular Energy

As discussed in chapter 6, adenosine triphosphate (ATP) is the unit of actual useable energy within our cells; food is broken down and absorbed through the digestive system, then sent to the body's cells where it is converted into ATP, which is often described as the correct currency of energy for the body. ATP provides the energy for nearly all biological functions, including growth, movement, detoxification, and electrical signals in nerves and the brain.

Like CoQ10, magnesium is essential for both the production and the storage of ATP.[68,69] Therefore, a deficiency in magnesium can also compromise energy production and the pumping ability of the heart. Indeed, magnesium deficiency has been indicated as an important contributing factor to heart failure.[70]

Scientists have suggested that magnesium's central role in the production of ATP can be traced back to the origins of life on earth, from magnesium's presence in the earth's crust (iron-magnesium silicate); to the primeval ocean being rich in magnesium; to the formation of chlorophyll, with magnesium in the center of the molecule-enabling photosynthesis; and eventually to the development of the animal cell containing magnesium-dependent ATP.[71,72]

Blood Pressure

Magnesium acts as a natural calcium channel blocker to reduce blood pressure, and it also corrects heart rhythm abnormalities. People with high blood pressure, angina, or arrhythmia (irregular heartbeat) are sometimes prescribed a medication known as a calcium channel blocker (CCB), one of the most widely used drugs in cardiovascular medicine.[73] CCBs reduce blood pressure through their action on smooth muscle cells. Smooth muscles, which are found in blood vessels, the gastrointestinal tract, and the bladder, provide slow rhythmic involuntary contractions. Figure 7.2 depicts a cross section of a blood vessel, showing the location of the smooth muscle within the wall of the blood vessel. When the smooth muscle contracts, the lumen (the internal diameter of the vessel) reduces, a necessary biological function in order to regulate circulation. CCBs exploit this mechanism in order to relax smooth muscles in people who have high blood pressure.

When calcium enters a smooth muscle cell, it interacts with contractile proteins to cause muscle contraction.[74] CCBs, as their name suggests, block calcium from entering the cell and therefore have a relaxing effect on blood vessels. However, magnesium has the same effect. Magnesium is a natural calcium channel blocker.

Magnesium, in many situations, counters the actions of calcium. Magnesium and calcium check and balance each other.[71] Calcium

elastica interna   endothelial cells   smooth muscle cells   lumen

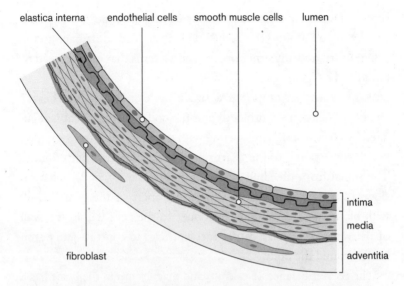

intima

media

fibroblast   adventitia

Figure 7.2. Cross section of a blood vessel showing the location of smooth muscle cells and the lumen. Image adapted from Drosenbach/Wikimedia Commons.

can be thought of as a stimulator, while magnesium is a calming or relaxing agent.

Studies going back almost a century have shown the blood pressure–lowering effects of magnesium.[75] And lower dietary intake of magnesium has been linked with higher blood pressure.[76–78] However, the circulation-improving actions of magnesium are not limited to its relaxation action on smooth muscle. Magnesium has also been shown, through various mechanisms, to improve the function of the endothelium (the cells that form the lining of blood vessels).[67,79,80]

Arrhythmia

The term arrhythmia refers to any problem with the rate or rhythm of the heartbeat, whether too fast, too slow, or with a fluctuating rhythm. Most arrhythmias are harmless, but some can be very serious. During an arrhythmia the heart might not be able to pump enough blood around the body,[81] which can lead to damage to the brain, heart, and any other organs and systems that are deprived of blood and oxygen.

A heartbeat encompasses a single cycle in which the heart's chambers relax and contract to pump blood. The heartbeat is regulated by electrical signals, starting with the sinus node (or SA node), which corresponds to the heart rate (number of beats per minute). The signal from the sinus node spreads to the AV node, where it slows to allow the ventricles (lower chambers of the heart) to fill with blood. The signal then continues to the cells within the wall of the ventricles, which causes the ventricles to contract and pump blood around the body.

The correct balance of calcium and magnesium in the heart has a stabilizing effect on this electrical activity,[71] and magnesium has been shown to be effective in treating many different forms of arrhythmia.[82,83]

The importance of magnesium in regulating the heartbeat is perhaps best concluded by the fact that Dr. Carolyn Dean, who has been researching magnesium for more than eighteen years, was awarded the Arrhythmia Alliance Outstanding Medical Contribution to Cardiac Rhythm Management Services Award in 2012, from the Heart Rhythm Society of the United Kingdom.[84]

Magnesium, Insulin, and Glucose

Magnesium plays an important role in glucose and insulin metabolism, by reducing insulin resistance and helping glucose enter into cells. People who have problems regulating blood glucose levels—in particular, people with type 2 diabetes or metabolic syndrome—have consistently been found to have lower levels of magnesium.

In one study, magnesium levels of people with metabolic syndrome were compared with those of healthy people. Of the 192 people with metabolic syndrome, 126 had low levels of magnesium in the blood, compared with just 19 of the 384 healthy people.[67,85]

Researchers at Harvard University looked at the dietary magnesium intake of approximately 85,000 women and 42,000 men, the results of which were published in the journal *Diabetes Care* in 2004. They found a correlation between type 2 diabetes and a lower dietary intake of magnesium.[86] The connection was still there even after adjusting the data to account for a large number of diabetes risk factors, such as weight and exercise levels, and other dietary factors that have been shown to be important, such as the glycemic load of the diet.

Of course, we should always be cautious about jumping to conclusions when an association is discovered; associations are often not actual causes. However, since we know that magnesium is involved in glucose metabolism, we can have more confidence that there is a valid biological mechanism.

Problems regulating blood glucose levels, and especially type 2 diabetes, pose major cardiovascular risks. Considering the worldwide epidemic of type 2 diabetes, anything that can be done to prevent problems associated with blood glucose dysregulation should be given some priority. But magnesium deficiency is another important factor currently completely ignored by health authorities.

Other Heart Benefits of Magnesium

People who have suffered a heart attack also have low blood levels of magnesium.[87–89] This seems to be most apparent in measurements of magnesium levels taken soon after a heart attack. After a period of around two weeks, blood magnesium levels seem to return to normal,[87] which could indicate that magnesium plays an important role in protecting heart muscle cells from dying.

At autopsy, the ventricular muscle of the heart contains less magnesium in patients who died of heart attack[90,91] compared with patients who died of other causes, and the actual infarcted tissue (the tissue that died because of a lack of blood and oxygen) contains even less magnesium. Disturbances in other minerals were also noted, including reductions in the amount of potassium and phosphorus.

Magnesium also has anticoagulation properties. When magnesium levels are low, the clotting action of calcium cannot be countered.[68,92]

In 2003, researchers published an article in the *American Heart Journal* that looked at the association between blood magnesium levels and adverse effects after coronary artery bypass graft surgery (CABG). The researchers examined the ability of blood magnesium levels to predict the incidence of heart attack and death. Up to one year after CABG, low blood levels of magnesium (below 4.4 mg/dL or 1.8 mmol/L) were associated with a twofold increased risk of death or heart attack.[93]

In short, magnesium is good for the heart and blood vessels because it plays a central role in cellular energy production, acts as a natural calcium channel blocker, improves the function of the endothelium and assists in vasodilation, is involved in glucose and insulin metabolism, regulates and stabilizes the heartbeat, and acts as an antagonist to calcium in other ways, including to prevent excessive blood clotting.

Magnesium Deficiency

Dr. Carolyn Dean suggests that 80 percent of people in the United States are deficient in magnesium.[68] Certainly, there is good reason to suspect widespread deficiency. In 2001–2002, 56 percent of the US population consumed less than the recommended amount of magnesium through their diet. By 2005–2006 the situation had improved a bit, with 48 percent of people not consuming enough magnesium.[94] However, there are a number of other important factors to consider concerning magnesium status.

Even if we eat lots of foods that contain higher amounts of magnesium (see tables 7.3 through 7.6), studies suggest that our foods do not contain as much magnesium as they used to. During the last seventy years or more, the way food is grown and prepared has changed dramatically in many countries, and the food available to us today has been shown to contain less nutrition than it used to. In 2002, foods contained, on average, 19 percent less magnesium than they did in 1940,[95] and many health practitioners believe things have since gotten worse.

Most diuretics (medications often prescribed for high blood pressure and various heart conditions) cause the body to lose some of its magnesium. In fact, just about anything that causes increased urination (for example, tea, coffee, or alcohol) also causes the body to lose magnesium.[96]

Table 7.3. Magnesium in Servings of Nuts and Seeds, from Most to Least

Nut or seed	Serving	Magnesium (in mg)
Pumpkin seeds	¼ cup	317
Brazil nuts	¼ cup	133
Sunflower seeds	¼ cup	119
Almonds	¼ cup	88–109
Cashews	¼ cup	90
Pine nuts	¼ cup	70–86
Flaxseeds	2 tbsp	78
Sesame seeds	2 tbsp	56–68
Peanuts	¼ cup	65
Chestnuts, Chinese	¼ cup	54
Peanut butter	2 tbsp	50–52
Hazelnuts	¼ cup	48–52

Table 7.4. Magnesium in Servings of Cooked Fish and Seafood, from Most to Least

Fish or seafood	Serving	Magnesium (in mg)
Salmon	75 g (2.5 oz.)	92
Halibut	75 g (2.5 oz.)	80
Mackerel	75 g (2.5 oz.)	73
Pollock	75 g (2.5 oz.)	64
Crab	75 g (2.5 oz.)	47

Table 7.5. Magnesium in Servings of Fruits and Vegetables, from Most to Least

Fruit or vegetable	Serving	Magnesium (in mg)
Prickly pear	1 fruit	88
Spinach, cooked	½ cup	83
Swiss chard, cooked	½ cup	80
Tamarind	½ cup	58
Potato (with skin), cooked	1 medium	47–52
Okra, cooked	½ cup	50

Table 7.6. Magnesium in Servings of Legumes, from Most to Least

Legume	Serving	Magnesium (in mg)
Black-eyed peas, cooked	¾ cup	121
Tempeh	¾ cup	116
Beans, cooked (black, lima, navy, adzuki, white kidney, pinto, great northern, chickpeas)	¾ cup	60–89
Lentils, cooked	¾ cup	52

As mentioned, magnesium is an antagonist to calcium, too much of which can result in the same problems as a magnesium deficiency. During the last few decades many people have actively increased the amount of dairy foods in their diet in order to increase their calcium intake, while others have taken calcium supplements. Dairy foods have a lot of calcium relative to magnesium; some doctors believe that too much dairy can create a magnesium deficiency.[96] Although the calcium content of foods has also declined because of food production methods, this has mostly applied to fruits and vegetables; the calcium content of dairy has not changed much.[109] Therefore, a significant number of people might now be consuming too much calcium relative to magnesium.

Various lifestyle factors relating to stress, strenuous exercise, and chronic illness can also contribute to the body's depletion of magnesium. In addition, according to Dr. Natasha Campbell-McBride, one molecule of sugar uses up twenty-eight molecules of magnesium.[38] Considering the astronomical increase in sugar consumption in many countries around the world during the last few decades, this is also likely to be a contributing factor to magnesium deficiency.

How can we find out if we are deficient in magnesium? As mentioned at the beginning of this chapter, only 1 percent of the body's magnesium is found in the blood, so blood tests for magnesium are not helpful (by themselves) for a lot of people. Generally, if the body's magnesium levels are very low, we would expect to see a low blood level. However, magnesium is taken from the tissues to maintain adequate levels in the blood, so a blood test could come back normal even though there is, in fact, a deficiency.

Health practitioners advocate a blood test along with an assessment of magnesium deficiency symptoms. Common symptoms include leg cramps, muscle twitches, muscle pain, fatigue and weakness, numbness or tingling, personality changes, heart palpitations, abnormal heart rhythms, and heart spasms. However, considering the number of biochemical actions in which magnesium plays a role, a deficiency can also affect many other functions of the body.

Magnesium Supplementation

Magnesium supplementation is beneficial for a huge number of people, and is something anyone with any kind of heart problem, high blood pressure, or diabetes should seriously consider. We should, however, always keep in mind that individuals react very differently to specific therapies, and anyone wishing to stop their blood pressure medication should do so with careful monitoring of their blood pressure while magnesium and any other supplements are introduced. It can take a few weeks or even a few months for magnesium levels to become optimal, and during this time it would be wise to gradually reduce any blood pressure medications, as appropriate (and, ideally, in consultation with a physician).

Magnesium supplements are also well-known to have a laxative effect. For anyone suffering with constipation, this might be a temporary added benefit, but loose stools for more than a few days are neither practical nor good for the body. Therefore, magnesium supplements have been developed that are more easily absorbed and are less likely to cause loose stools. Alternatively, magnesium can be absorbed through the skin by taking a bath in Epson salt (magnesium sulfate), and magnesium sprays are also available.

Oral magnesium supplements should be avoided in cases of low stomach acid, as magnesium has an alkalizing effect. In cases of weak digestion associated with low stomach acid production, magnesium could disrupt the acid/alkaline base of the stomach. The acidity of the stomach is important not only for digestion but also as a defense against microbes. If the stomach is not sufficiently acid, this part of the immune system can be affected, or digestion can be made worse, by oral magnesium. Anyone with poor kidney function, kidney disease, very low heart rate, or bowel obstruction should avoid magnesium supplements.

Magnesium Injections

In 1963, Dr. S. E. Browne, a general practitioner from England, wrote a letter to the British Medical Journal[97] about the benefits of using magnesium for the prevention and treatment of heart disease. In his letter, Dr. Browne cited a number of studies done in the 1950s where magnesium injections had been shown to be extremely beneficial to cardiac patients.

Dr. Browne wrote:

> Over a period of two and a half years in my own general practice I have found magnesium sulphate (intramuscularly or in resistant cases intravenously) to be by far the most powerful vasodilator available in all types of peripheral or cardiac vascular disease.

For the next thirty years, Dr. Browne continued to administer magnesium sulphate, summarizing this work in an article published in the Journal of Nutritional Medicine in 1994,[98] including the outcomes for different patient groups. For angina, 126 patients were treated with intravenous magnesium sulphate, 116 of whom were either completely relieved of pain or markedly improved.

For heart attack patients, good recovery in all 59 patients treated with magnesium sulphate was seen without any evidence of arrhythmias (which normally affect about 90 percent of people after a heart attack).[99] Dr. Browne also stated that the major part of the benefits were attributable to the magnesium sulphate opening up collateral circulation within the heart.

Around the same time, other studies also showed that magnesium injections benefited cardiac patients.[100–102] This included a larger study published in *The Lancet*[100] where the researchers concluded:

> Intravenous magnesium sulphate is a simple, safe, and widely applicable treatment. Its efficacy in reducing early mortality of myocardial infarction [heart attack] is comparable to, but independent of, that of thrombolytic or antiplatelet therapy.

And another study, published in the *International Journal of Cardiology*,[103] concluded:

> These results suggest that magnesium administration reduces the incidence of serious tachyarrhythmias and death after acute myocardial infarction and that this simple regime warrants further study.

Until the mid-1990s, almost all of the published studies had shown magnesium injections to be beneficial. So, for a while things were looking good for magnesium sulphate therapy. Then, in 1995 a large study was published in the *Lancet* that involved more than 58,000 patients.[104] This study, named the ISIS-4 Study, concluded that there was no benefit associated with magnesium sulphate injections and, in fact, the injections caused slight harm.

However, Dr. Damien Downing, president of the British Society for Ecological Medicine, has since published an article describing how the researchers of the ISIS-4 Study overdosed the patients by giving possibly too much magnesium sulphate, at the wrong time, and administered it both too quickly and in an uncontrolled way.[105] Obviously, giving too much magnesium too quickly will cause very low blood pressure and associated complications. Dr. Downing argued that this overdosing could have been avoided if the understanding gained from the previous studies had been incorporated into the ISIS-4 Study.

Sodium and Potassium

Various health authorities tell us that consuming too much salt is bad for the heart. More specifically, experts are concerned about the intake of sodium compared with potassium. The World Health Organization advises adults to consume less than 5 grams of salt, less than 2 grams of sodium, and more than 3.5 grams of potassium each day.[106]

The concern is largely based on observations that a high sodium intake, or a low potassium intake relative to sodium, can increase blood pressure. The American Heart Association has even stricter guidance and recommends an intake of no more than 1.5 grams of sodium per day.[107] This guidance is based on studies that have suggested that sodium intake below this level is associated with lower blood pressure. The mechanisms by which sodium intake influences blood pressure are not yet fully understood, but they are thought to be related primarily to the intimate relationship between sodium and water.

When sodium is absorbed through the gastrointestinal tract, it brings water with it, keeping the body hydrated. The major fluids of the body are sustained because of sodium. Without sodium the fluid component of blood and the fluids that surround the body's cells would lose their water, leading to dehydration and death.

The body uses various systems to try to keep the correct balance of sodium and water. Information is sent from the blood vessels and the brain that tells the kidneys to retain sodium or excrete sodium in the urine. Sodium intake also causes changes in thirst as a means of regulating water relative to sodium.

If too much sodium is consumed, sodium's affinity with water is believed to cause an increase in the fluid volume and an increase in the pressure within the blood vessels. Potassium does not have the same affinity with water. In fact, potassium and sodium are antagonistic to each other; potassium counters the effects of sodium, and vice versa.

The intracellular space (inside the body's cells) contains a lot more potassium than the extracellular space (the fluid surrounding the body's cells) and the reverse is true for sodium. Therefore, the body clearly requires an appropriate balance of sodium and potassium, but the current recommendations for sodium intake might not be serving us well.

Studies on salt intake are somewhat problematic. Comparing data between various studies is difficult because two different methods are used for measuring salt intake: measuring urinary sodium excretion and estimating dietary intake. Twenty-four-hour urinary sodium excretion might be the most accurate method, since 90–95 percent of sodium intake is excreted in the urine. However, it is not practical to collect twenty-four-hour's worth of urine, particularly during an extended study period, so researchers have suggested that fasting morning urine is a reliable substitute.[108,109] Urinary sodium excretion does not account for sodium loss due to sweat.

Dietary intake is measured with the aid of food diaries and questionnaires. However, there is considerable room for inaccuracies if the study participant does not recall all of the foods they consumed. Further inaccuracies can arise because of differences in the sodium content of common foods and if table salt is not included in the analysis. In addition, portion size needs to be accurately accounted for.[108]

Dietary recommendations for salt intake are largely based on clinical studies that use urinary analysis. But population surveys have used dietary recall for the analysis, and there is no existing method for comparing these two different measurements.[108]

The analysis is made more complicated by differences in how each person consumes sodium. One person might have a higher sodium intake because of consuming processed foods such as ready-made meals, whereas another person might be getting their sodium from a more balanced diet that also includes more fresh fruit and vegetables. Therefore, some diets might be high in sodium but also high in potassium. Some people's diets could also be high in other cardio-protective nutrients that could be offsetting the otherwise negative impact of the sodium.

Notwithstanding these difficulties in interpreting the data, studies have generally, on balance, shown a connection between lower sodium intake and lower blood pressure,[110–116] although the reduction in blood pressure associated with lower sodium intake is often quite small. For example, an analysis completed by the Cochrane Hypertension Group found that a modest reduction in sodium intake resulted in an average reduction of 5 mmHg in systolic blood pressure and a reduction of 2.7 mmHg in diastolic blood pressure for people with high blood pressure.[116] People with normal blood pressure had smaller reductions (2.3 mmHg for systolic and 1 mmHg for diastolic). Mathematically, if a 2 mmHg reduction in diastolic blood pressure is applied across a very large population (such as nationwide), this would result in an overall 6 percent reduction in heart disease risk.[117] But how relevant these small reductions in blood pressure are for individual people is debatable.

Since blood pressure fluctuates as a result of a wide range of different conditions, it is important to look for a connection between lower sodium intake and an actual reduction in cardiovascular problems, rather than looking at changes in blood pressure alone. Such studies have had mixed results; some have confirmed an increased risk of cardiovascular disease in connection with a high sodium intake,[118–121] while others have not.[122–125] In fact, overall, researchers have suggested that the relationship between sodium intake and cardiovascular disease follows a J-shaped curve[110] whereby both a low and high sodium intake could involve an increased risk.

Statistically, the lowest cardiovascular risks have been seen with a sodium intake of 3–5 grams per day, with an increased risk associated with both higher levels (above 5 grams per day) and lower levels (below 3 grams per day).[110] This is important because although the data does confirm some kind of connection with sodium intake, the current recommendations are set too low and are associated with an increased risk. As mentioned above, health authorities currently recommend a sodium intake of 1.5–2 grams per day. Overall, this level of intake is associated with an increase in cardiovascular problems.

Health authorities could have become blinded by the blood pressure–lowering effect of a very low-sodium diet, and they could have failed to consider the other effects of such a diet. A very low-sodium diet has been shown to alter levels of some hormones and cytokines that are involved in cell-to-cell communication.[110,126] A moderate, rather than low, sodium intake has even been shown to improve outcomes for some heart failure patients.[126]

As mentioned, we should also consider potassium intake, not just sodium intake, as there is some evidence that potassium might exhibit a similar relationship. A study that analyzed the data from approximately 39,000 patients in the United States who had already suffered a heart attack found a U-shaped curve. Similar to sodium, both low and high levels of potassium were associated with an increased cardiovascular risk, with the lowest risk associated with moderate potassium levels.[127]

The J-shaped and U-shaped curves for sodium and potassium respectively might be a further indication that the levels relative to each other are what is most important. Indeed, there is some data suggesting that a higher sodium-to-potassium excretion ratio is more strongly associated with increased cardiovascular risk than that of sodium or potassium alone.[128,125]

Sodium/Potassium Balance after Heart Attack

The importance of the correct balance of sodium and potassium is further illustrated by the observation of heart muscle tissue after a heart attack. In an acute heart attack, tissue damage can be seen in three zones of heart muscle tissue. The core area consists of necrotic tissue and dead cells due to the absence of oxygen. Next to this there is an area of severe injury that is composed of cells that will die if the metabolic derangement cannot be corrected. Last, surrounding this area is a less ischemic zone, where cellular function is impaired but is reversible. In short, there is a gradient of extent of damage and metabolic derangement, with the extent of damage gradually reducing with increasing distance away from the necrotic core.

The damage gradient correlates with the amount of sodium inside the cell. As mentioned, there is a lot more sodium outside the cell (the extracellular space) than inside the cell. Under healthy conditions, there is a powerful mechanism for constantly pumping excess sodium out of the cell, the sodium-potassium pump; however, after a heart attack the membrane of the cell is damaged and additional sodium enters the cell. The excess sodium increases the fluid volume of the cell, causing it to swell, and cellular function and the ability to pump the excess sodium out of the cell is impaired.

The outer area of tissue damage typically corresponds with a 50 percent increase in the amount of sodium in the cell. The intermediate zone corresponds with a 200 percent increase in sodium, and the inner necrotic core has a 300 percent increase in sodium.

At the same time a similar, but reverse, situation is observed with potassium. Normally there is much more potassium inside the cell than outside, but after a heart attack there is a decrease in the potassium content inside the cell that again corresponds with the degree of tissue damage within the three affected zones.

These observations led Dr. Demetrio Sodi Pallares of Mexico City to develop a polarizing solution to help correct the sodium-potassium deregulation after an acute heart attack. The solution was based on earlier work done by Henry Laborit, a French researcher, and consisted of glucose, insulin, and potassium. The insulin helps the glucose and potassium into the cell.

Dr. Pallares had quite dramatic positive results using the polarizing solution in the 1960s, and a number of prominent cardiologists around the world also started administering it.[129] At that time, and in a number of studies completed since, the polarizing solution reduced the number of deaths, the amount of tissue damage, and complications such as arrhythmias after a heart attack.[130-141]

In fact, the potential benefits of the polarizing solution also extend into other areas of medicine that are beyond the scope of this book and involve the electrical potential across the cell membrane and the additional use of electromagnetic fields. A more detailed discussion is available in the excellent book *Bioelectromagnetic and Subtle Energy Medicine*.[129]

Conclusion

So what does this mean for the millions of people trying to consume a diet that is good for the heart? Clearly, the amount of sodium consumed relative to potassium is important. On average, people in the United States, for example, consume 3.4 grams of sodium each day.[142] The American public has repeatedly been told that this is more than double the recommended amount. However, the data from the studies mentioned in this chapter suggests that this level of consumption is not harmful. But at the same time, there is reason to think that potassium intake might be too low compared with sodium intake.

Many countries around the world now consume more processed foods, which often contain sodium as a preservative. This inherently means that people are also consuming fewer fresh vegetables and fruit, the foods that contain high levels of potassium. So, although sodium intake by itself might not be cause for concern, it is likely that the balance of sodium to potassium might not be ideal for a lot of people.

Therefore, the best, easiest, and most effective solution for most people is to simply reduce consumption of processed food in favor of more fresh vegetables and fruit, which will, of course, provide additional nutritional benefits (see tables 7.7 through 7.9). Driving down sodium intake alone could be harmful, since there is a danger of becoming deficient in sodium.

This simple approach applies to the majority of people who do not have a diagnosed heart problem and have a well-functioning

Table 7.7. Potassium in Servings of Vegetables, from Most to Least

Vegetable	Serving	Potassium (in mg)
Beet greens, boiled	1 cup	1,309
Potato, baked	1 medium	1,081
Sweet potato, cooked	1 medium	694
Parsnip, cooked	1 cup	573
Beets, boiled	1 cup	519
Brussels sprouts, cooked	1 cup	495
Winter squash, baked	1 cup	494
Broccoli, cooked	1 cup	457
Carrot, raw	1 cup	352
Artichoke, cooked	1 medium	343
Tomato	1 medium	292
Okra, cooked	1 cup	216

Table 7.8. Potassium in Servings of Fruit, from Most to Least

Fruit	Serving	Potassium (in mg)
Cantaloupe	1 cup	427
Banana	1 medium	422
Apricots, dried	10 halves	407
Grapefruit	1 medium	332
Prunes	5	307
Nectarine	1 medium	273
Dates	5	272
Raisins (seedless)	¼ cup	271
Strawberries	1 cup	254
Blackberries	1 cup	233

Table 7.9. Potassium in Servings of Additional Foods, from Most to Least

Food	Serving	Potassium (in mg)
Lentils, cooked	3 oz.	731
Salmon, baked	3 oz.	347
Ground beef, broiled	3 oz.	258
Turkey, roasted	3 oz.	212
Almonds	24	200

sodium-potassium pump. However, anyone with an existing heart condition or other medical problem might need to more carefully control their sodium and potassium balance and should certainly discuss this with their physician. In these cases, hopefully, the information contained in this chapter will enable more informed discussions with medical professionals.

Water

According to an alien race encountered by the starship *Enterprise* on the television series *Star Trek: The Next Generation*, humans are "ugly bags of mostly water."[143] Although meant for entertainment purposes, the statement is basically accurate. By volume, two thirds of our cells' contents are water, but because the water molecule is so small, lots of water molecules are needed to constitute two-thirds volume. In fact, calculated in terms of the number of molecules, 99 percent of our body's molecules are water molecules. It is then perhaps not a huge surprise that hydration status can affect the heart.

In 2002, researchers published a study that investigated the amount of water consumed each day and the number of heart disease deaths in the United States.[144] The study included around 20,000 men and women between the ages of thirty-eight and one hundred, who were followed for six years. The researchers found a strong correlation between increased water consumption and a reduction in heart disease deaths. On average, people who drank five or more glasses of water per day had about half the risk of dying of heart disease compared with people who drank two glasses or less per day (see figure 7.3). The association remained the same even after eliminating a wide range of other factors such as age, smoking status, high blood pressure, body mass index, education level, and estrogen replacement therapy in menopausal women.

None of the people included in this study showed any prior signs of heart disease, so for many people in the study, their baseline risk was already low. However, these are still dramatic results in favor of probably the simplest intervention possible: drinking more water. In addition, the results indicate that optimum water intake could be more effective at reducing heart disease mortality than statin medications.

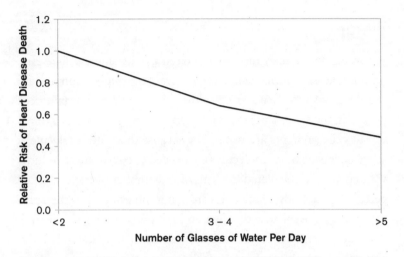

Figure 7.3. The relationship between the number of 8 oz. (250 ml) glasses of water consumed per day compared with the risk of dying of heart disease. Graph shown includes the data for men. Adapted from Chan J, Knutsen SF, Blix GG, Lee JW, Fraser GE. Water, other fluids, and fatal coronary heart disease: the Adventist Health Study. *Am J Epidemiol.* 2002;155(9):827–833.

Water consumption is not included in any of the cardiovascular risk calculators that doctors use. Current clinical guidelines encourage doctors to look for markers that have corresponding medications that can be used to treat them. Globally, hundreds of billions of dollars have been spent on statins during the last two decades, and that does not include the financial and health costs associated with the adverse effects of statins. On the other hand, drinking water is practically free, and its only side effects are improved health in other areas.

As with the interpretation of all studies, we have to be careful about confusing associations with actual causes. Association does not prove causation. So, in addition to the data, we should always ask if there is a plausible biological mechanism.

The cardiovascular benefits of drinking water are at least in part due to improvements in blood viscosity and blood-clotting factors. Increased blood viscosity (an increased general thickness and stickiness of the blood) is well known to increase the risk of heart disease.[144–154] Blood viscosity is a direct measure of the ability of the blood to flow through the vessels; it determines how much friction the blood causes against the vessels and how hard the heart has to work in order to pump blood and oxygen to organs and tissues. Blood viscosity is therefore a key aspect of heart disease. Although water intake is not the only factor that can affect blood viscosity, it certainly is one of the factors.[155–157]

It is well known within the medical community that heart attacks often happen in the morning; notably, blood viscosity is also often greater in the morning.[144,158,159] During the night, fluid levels are not topped up as they are during the day, which could be one factor accounting for increased viscosity and increased heart attacks in the morning.[144]

Drinks that have a mild diuretic effect, such as caffeinated drinks, can also increase blood viscosity due to fluid loss.[160]

Electrolyte Balance

Dehydration can also affect the body's electrolyte balance. Electrolytes are minerals in the body that have an electric charge. Sodium, calcium, magnesium, potassium, chlorine, and phosphate all act as electrolytes; these are used by the cells to maintain voltages across their membranes and carry electrical impulses.

These electrical impulses, or signals, are critical for the function of the heart. The heart cells use electrolytes to maintain the proper electrical signal that forms the basis of the heartbeat. If the electrolyte balance is disturbed because of dehydration, this can affect the rhythm of the heart, causing arrhythmia.

Of course, too much water intake can also disturb the balance of electrolytes, so we should aim for our individual optimum level of intake.

Hard Water

Whether water is considered hard or soft is determined by its mineral content. Hard water contains more minerals, especially calcium and magnesium, than soft water. Since the late 1950s researchers have suggested that people who drink hard water have a lower incidence of cardiovascular deaths,[161,162] and this hypothesis has been supported by a number of studies,[163–168] with the most important factor seeming to be magnesium content.

Magnesium deficiency is one of the most important nutritional factors associated with heart disease, as discussed earlier in this chapter, and studies have shown that waterborne magnesium is absorbed about 30 percent more efficiently than the magnesium obtained from food.[168] Drinking hard water is an excellent way to top up magnesium intake and prevent a deficiency, and hence help prevent heart disease.

Precautions

As noted, it is possible to have too much water. As with everything else, individuals have unique requirements for water. Heart failure patients, in particular, need to carefully regulate their fluid intake, since too much water can increase demands on the heart. Heart failure patients should consult with their doctor to determine optimum fluid intake.

CHAPTER EIGHT

Conclusion: What to Do

The main thesis of this book is that heart disease is caused by the complex interaction of a large number of factors, and therefore, an individual person's risk of heart attack cannot be reduced to a simple risk calculator. The risk calculator in current use serves the purposes of the pharmaceutical companies; it focuses specifically on suggested risk factors that medications exist to modify.

Heart disease is caused by the interaction of factors associated with the stress response, nutrition, lifestyle, the immune system, and the environment. Not only do all of these categories interact, but the importance of each category varies greatly between different people. For example, one person's heart attack could be caused primarily by psychological stress, which predisposed that person to infection. Another person's heart attack could be caused by a combination of nutritional deficiencies and high blood glucose levels.

Taking a statin, or any other medication, offers very little protection against any of the real causes of heart attacks. The data from statin clinical trials predicts that statins could prevent a heart attack for around 1.6 percent of people who take the medication over a five-year time period.[1] But we must also keep in mind that although this data comes mostly from randomized clinical trials, these trials have inherent weaknesses.

The populations used in clinical trials are selected, and the trial procedure involves a "run-in period" during which large numbers of trial participants can be excluded from the final analysis, for a variety of reasons decided by the researchers. The trial itself can be designed in a way that is more likely to result in a positive result for the medication being tested, and the final published report is written by statisticians and professional writers who work for the company sponsoring the trial. Overall, it could be argued that clinical trial reports do not accurately represent the real-life populations who are expected to take the medications. In fact, when researchers look retrospectively at the benefits of statins, statins appear to be having no positive impact.[2] In order to prevent heart disease and heart attacks, the most important factors to consider are summarized below.

Stress Management/Relaxation

We have seen how excess negative stress can have a profound effect on the heart; it can change the condition of the heart itself, the electrical control of the heartbeat, and the health of the coronary arteries. When the body is under chronic negative stress, essential nutrients get used up more quickly than they can be replenished, weakening the immune system and making the body even more susceptible to disease. Therefore, stress management and relaxation are a critical part of any heart disease prevention plan.

Relaxation is individual in exactly the same way that stress is. What one person finds relaxing, another person might find stressful. Some people love to take a vacation at a beach resort with nothing to do but recline by the ocean or the pool and read a book, whereas other people prefer to go trekking in the mountains. Both can be equally relaxing and energizing, as long as they fit with the individual.

Most people know what relaxes them. However, there is a distinction between relaxing activities and activities that merely distract. For example, watching television might be thought of as relaxing, but it depends on what is being watched. Often, watching television is a distraction rather than a relaxation activity. We must be vigilant about what actually makes us feel more relaxed afterward. If we do not feel noticeably more relaxed after the activity, then the activity has been a mere distraction.

Meditation is up to eleven times more beneficial than taking a statin medication, and the only side effects associated with meditation are better clarity of thought and improved overall sense of well-being. In essence, for stress reduction, we are looking for activities that nourish the parasympathetic nervous system (PNS). In addition to meditation, deep breathing, time spent in nature, playing with children or animals, yoga, tai chi, chi kung, and sexual activity—all these also nurture the parasympathetic nervous system.

Monitor Waist Circumference

This book has not included a detailed discussion of obesity, partly because several excellent books already exist that investigate its causes in considerable detail[3–5] and also because where heart disease is concerned, obesity is a symptom that things are going in the wrong direction in terms of other factors. A low-fat/high-carbohydrate diet is more likely to cause weight gain,[6–13] and, as was mentioned in chapter 5, stress causes central obesity, or an increase in visceral fat.

Experts and health authorities still use body mass index (BMI) when determining if someone is overweight, and BMI is also used in some of the cardiovascular risk calculators. BMI is a crude measure of weight compared with height, and it can produce some misleading measurements. For example, if someone who is not very tall has

a lot of muscle, their BMI can put them in the obese category even
though they have a very low percentage of body fat. In addition,
BMI does not tell us how much fat is subcutaneous fat and how
much is central obesity/visceral fat, the latter being of more rele-
vance to cardiovascular health.

Central obesity/visceral fat is associated with the metabolic
abnormalities that lead to type 2 diabetes. On average, increased
central obesity more than doubles the risk for type 2 diabetes,[14] and
people with type 2 diabetes have the same risk of heart attack as
people who have already had a heart attack.[15]

An accurate measurement of visceral fat involves a medical scan
that is expensive, impractical, and out of reach for most people. However, a simple measurement of waist circumference can be useful. For
most people, knowing waist circumference is probably more useful
than knowing BMI. To measure waist circumference (using a tape
measure) start at the top of the hip bone, then bring the tape measure
all the way around, level with the navel. The tape should not be too
tight or twisted, and the stomach should be in a neutral position. For
men, waist circumference should ideally be 40 inches or less, and for
women 35 inches or less. When waist circumference starts to creep
up higher, the risk for metabolic diseases, particularly type 2 diabetes,
starts to significantly increase. However, skinny people can also have a
large amount of visceral fat, while appearing to be slim on the outside.

Exercise

We all know that exercise strengthens the cardiovascular system
and protects us from heart disease. In fact, general fitness is strongly
associated with protection from dying of all causes. People with the
lowest capacity for exercise have 4.5 times the risk of dying when
compared with people who have the greatest capacity for exercise.[16]

Exercise does not have to take place in a gym. Any kind of physical movement that increases the heart rate is likely to be beneficial. Health authorities recommend at least thirty minutes of movement or exercise on as many days during the week as possible.

Exercise is also very beneficial for people with diabetes and for the prevention of diabetes, because exercise increases insulin sensitivity[17] (insulin resistance is the hallmark of diabetes). Exercise also helps to reduce visceral fat. This should be a source of encouragement for people who struggle to lose weight when exercising. The harmful visceral fat could still be reducing even if the number on the scale does not change very much. Waist circumference is a better indicator than a bathroom scale.

However, as with everything, it is possible to have too much of a good thing, even exercise. If one exercises too much without adequate recovery time, the parasympathetic nervous system becomes suppressed in a way that is similar to that of a chronic stress situation. In chapter 5 we described how the stress response encourages the heart to rely on the sugar-burning energy system and, as a result, the heart can become damaged due to the resulting acidosis. In one study, researchers analyzed the blood of collapsed Boston marathon runners. Compared with asymptomatic runners, the collapsed runners had disturbances in electrolytes (low levels of ionized calcium and magnesium) and high levels of lactic acid. In fact, acidosis was found in 95 percent of the collapsed runners.[18]

Nutrition

Nutrition can be incredibly complicated, with nutritionists offering many conflicting viewpoints and opinions. In addition, as individuals we have precise individual nutritional requirements. However, in general, the basis of cardio-protective nutrition can be quite straightforward.

Animal based proteins (meat, fish, seafood, poultry, and eggs) provide the best nutritional source for vitamins A, D, B_1, B_2, B_3, B_6, B_{12}, pantothenic acid, biotin, coenzyme Q10, and saturated fatty acids, but these foods do not contain vitamin C, which humans need to consume every day. Vitamin C is provided by vegetables and fruit. Potassium, another important nutrient for the heart, is also obtained from vegetables. Therefore, ideally, humans should consume both animal- and plant-based foods every day.

Vegetables should be the main carbohydrate that is consumed, since vegetables do not cause the same dramatic fluctuations in blood glucose as other carbohydrates. In particular, there is evidence that cruciferous vegetables are particularly good for the heart.

There is currently a raging debate about the nutritional adequacy of a vegetarian diet. If the animal proteins that are consumed largely consist of factory-farmed animals that are routinely injected with hormones and antibiotics and fed foods that they were not designed to eat (such as cows being fed grain instead of grass), then there is a strong argument to be made for a vegetarian diet being healthier, but it is not because of the fat or cholesterol content of animal-based foods.

Meat, poultry, and eggs from organic farms, and wild fish and seafood (not withstanding the way humans have polluted the oceans) are highly nutritious and cardio-protective.

And of course there are a number of possible compromises, such as following a largely vegetarian diet that includes fish and eggs. Whether or not a vegetarian diet supplies all of the required nutrients depends on the individual person and their lifestyle.

It is also a good idea to consume fermented foods whenever possible. "Fermented" simply means that the food is left to sit until the sugars and carbohydrates convert into health-promoting bacteria. Fermented foods could support the digestive system and the immune system, and they also contain vitamin K_2, which helps calcium enter into the bones where it is needed and, in theory, can help to keep calcium away from the coronary arteries where it might otherwise accumulate and cause hardening and stiffening.

Many traditional cultures that are known for their high level of nutrition and good health consume fermented foods. One obvious example is the Japanese, who regularly consume pickles and miso soup. In some parts of Japan they regularly eat the fermented food called natto, which contains incredibly high levels of vitamin K_2.

Nutritional Supplements

Many people are deficient in **CoQ10**; CoQ10 supplementation has been shown to reduce the risk of heart problems and death from heart disease. Some data suggest that CoQ10 supplementation is six times more effective than statins, and without any adverse effects. Between the two forms of CoQ10, some evidence suggests that ubiquinol could be more beneficial than ubiquinone; this could be especially important for the elderly and for anyone with a chronic medical condition. In general, studies that have shown considerable benefit have used a dosage of between 120 and 600 mg per day of CoQ10. Since not all of the CoQ10 can be absorbed in one go, it is better to spread the dose out into two or three times during the day to maximize the absorption. One hundred milligrams of ubiquinol twice per day is probably a good place to start for most people. CoQ10 is also best taken with food containing fat or oil.

Some studies have shown that **omega-3** supplementation can reduce the risk of suffering a heart attack. So far, the results have not been anywhere near the level of results that have been seen with CoQ10 supplementation; however, omega-3 supplementation could be more beneficial than taking a statin medication.

Magnesium supplementation is beneficial for a large number of people and, in particular, is certainly something to seriously consider for anyone with any kind of heart problem, high blood pressure, or diabetes. However, there are a few things to consider before taking magnesium supplements (see chapter 7).

Supplemental **vitamin C** at a dosage of up to 1 gram per day should be considered, with a higher dosage for people with a diagnosed heart problem or type 2 diabetes.

A general multivitamin and multimineral supplement could also be beneficial and could aid absorption of the other specific nutrients. Many nutritionists have the opinion that whole food–based nutritional supplements are more beneficial. Most supplements still consist of synthetically derived chemicals, but food state or whole food–based supplements are manufactured from real foods. Some health practitioners believe that these whole food–based supplements contain other ingredients in tiny amounts that are naturally present in foods and aid the assimilation of nutrients. Because of the potential for better assimilation, whole food–based supplements can usually be taken at a lower dosage than their synthetic equivalents.

Environmental Influences

Environmental influences can be difficult to manage. However, it is still worth keeping this factor in mind when deciding to move to a new location or country. One pollutant that can certainly be managed is cigarette smoking.

Cigarette smoking is a universally accepted and well-known cause of heart disease. Large reductions in cardiovascular deaths have been seen in countries where large numbers of people have stopped smoking.[19] Although health authorities regularly advise people to stop smoking (as they should), the authorities hardly ever mention the actual mechanisms associated with how cigarette smoking causes heart disease. Smoking cigarettes causes the same changes in the autonomic nervous system that were discussed as associated with the stress response, specifically the activation of the sympathetic nervous system and the down regulation of the para-sympathetic nervous system.[20,21]

––––––––––

There is a great opportunity for the future of heart disease prevention to be based on a more integrated approach that considers a wide range of the real causes of heart disease as discussed and that is tailored to the individual person. Studies have shown a number of nutritional interventions to be superior to statins in both efficacy and the safety profile. Redirecting resources to these areas and stress management is highly likely to be of much greater benefit to society than the continuation of the prescription of statin medication en masse.

NOTES

Introduction

1. Ioannidis JPA. More than a billion people taking statins? Potential implications of the new cardiovascular guidelines. *JAMA*. 2014;311(5):463.

2. Researchers often use the number needed to treat (NNT) as one
way of measuring the effectiveness of a medication. This will be
described in more detail in chapter 4. The NNT for statin medications in primary prevention is continuously updated and available.
The NNT. http://www.thennt.com/nnt/statins-for-heart-disease
-prevention-without-prior-heart-disease. Accessed March 15, 2017.

3. Rifkin E, Bouwer E. *The illusion of certainty*. New York: Springer; 2007.

4. Smith J. *Statin nation: the great cholesterol cover-up* [DVD]. 2012.

5. Smith J. *Statin nation II: what really causes heart disease* [DVD]. 2015.

6. Lenzer J. Majority of panelists on controversial new cholesterol
guideline have current or recent ties to drug manufacturers. *BMJ*.
2013;347:f6989.

7. American College of Cardiology, American Heart Association.
ASCVD risk estimator. http://tools.acc.org/ASCVD-Risk-Estimator.
Accessed March 15, 2017.

8. Kolata G. Risk calculator for cholesterol appears flawed. *New York
Times*, November 17, 2013.

9. Scherstén T, Rosch PJ, Arfors KE, Sundberg R. The cholesterol hypothesis: time for the obituary? *Scand Cardiovasc J*. 2011;45(6):322–323.

10. Hamazaki T, Okuyama H, Ogushi Y, Hama R. Towards a paradigm
shift in cholesterol treatment. A re-examination of the cholesterol
issue in japan. *Ann Nutr Metab*. 2015;66(suppl 4):1–116.

11. Ravnskov U, Diamond DM, Hama R, et al. Lack of an association or
an inverse association between low-density-lipoprotein cholesterol and
mortality in the elderly: a systematic review. *BMJ Open*. 2016;6:e010401.

12. Ravnskov U. *The cholesterol myths.* White Plains, MD: NewTrends Publishing; 2000.

13. Kendrick M. *The great cholesterol con.* London: John Blake Publishing; 2008.

14. Ravnskov U, DiNicolantonio JJ, Harcombe Z, et al. The questionable benefits of exchanging saturated fat with polyunsaturated fat. *Mayo Clin Proc.* 2014;89(4):451–453.

15. Hamazaki T, Okuyama H, Ogushi Y, Hama R. Cholesterol issues in Japan—why are the goals of cholesterol levels set so low? *Ann Nutr Metab.* 2013;62(1):32–36.

16. Sultan S, Hynes N. The ugly side of statins. Systematic appraisal of the contemporary un-known unknowns. *Open J Endocr Metab Dis.* 2013;3(3):179–185.

17. Canto JG, Kiefe CI, Rogers WJ, et al. Number of coronary heart disease risk factors and mortality in patients with first myocardial infarction. *JAMA.* 2011;306(19):2120–2127.

Chapter One: The Etiology of Heart Disease

1. British Heart Foundation. High cholesterol. https://www.bhf.org.uk/heart-health/risk-factors/high-cholesterol. Accessed March 15, 2017.

2. Barnes B, Barnes C. *Solved: the riddle of heart attacks.* Fort Collins, CO: Robinson Press; 1976.

3. Anitschkow N. Experimental arteriosclerosis in animals. In: Cowdry EV. *Arteriosclerosis: A survey of the problem.* New York: Macmillan; 1933.

4. Friedland IB. Investigations on the influence of thyroid preparations on experimental hypercholesterolemia and atherosclerosis. *Z Ges Exp Med.* 1933;87:683–695.

5. Keys A. Atherosclerosis: a problem in newer public health. *J Mt Sinai Hosp N Y.* 1953;20(2):118–139.

6. Ravnskov U. *The cholesterol myths.* White Plains, MD: NewTrends Publishing; 2000.

7. Allender S, Scarborough P, Peto V, Kaur A, Rayner M. Coronary heart disease statistics. London: British Heart Foundation; 2008.

8. Capewell S, Ford ES. Why have total cholesterol levels declined in most developed countries? *BMC Public Health.* 2011;11:641.

9. Kaunitz H. Cholesterol and repair processes in arteriosclerosis. *Lipids*.1978;13(5):373–374.

10. Kaunitz H. Dietary lipids and arteriosclerosis. *J Am Oil Chem Soc.* 1975;52(8):293–297.

11. Sachdeva A, Cannon CP, Deedwania PC, et al. Lipid levels in patients hospitalized with coronary artery disease: an analysis of 136,905 hospitalizations in Get With The Guidelines. *Am Heart J.* 2009;157(1):111–117.

12. Carroll MD, Lacher DA, Sorlie PD, et al. Trends in serum lipids and lipoproteins of adults, 1960–2002. *JAMA.* 2005;294(14):1773–1781.

13. For comparison, the LDL level of people twenty years and older was used. However, women around the same age as those included in the *American Heart Journal* study had an LDL level of 133 and men around the same age had an LDL level of 127 mg/dL—which means that in real terms, the difference was even more significant. The average level of LDL cholesterol for American adults age twenty and older in 2010 was 116 mg/dL. Mann D. Cholesterol levels down among U.S. adults. *Web MD.* October 16, 2012. http://www.webmd .com/cholesterol-management/news/20121016/cholesterol-levels -down-adults#1. Accessed March 10, 2017.

14. Cheng KH, Chu CS, Lin TH, Lee KT, Sheu SH, Lai WT. Lipid paradox in acute myocardial infarction—the association with 30-day in-hospital mortality. *Crit Care Med.* 2015;43(6):1255–1264.

15. Al-Mallah MH, Hatahet H, Cavalcante JL, Khanal S. Low admission LDL-cholesterol is associated with increased 3-year all-cause mortality in patients with non ST segment elevation myocardial infarction. *Cardiol J.* 2009;16(3):227–233.

16. Smith J. *Statin nation II: what really causes heart disease* [DVD]. 2015.

17. Smith J. *$29 billion reasons to lie about cholesterol.* Troubador: 2009.

18. Hamazaki T, Okuyama H, Ogushi Y, Hama R. Towards a paradigm shift in cholesterol treatment. A re-examination of the cholesterol issue in japan. *Ann Nutr Metab.* 2015;66(suppl 4):1–116.

19. Ravnskov U, Diamond DM, Hama R, et al. Lack of an association or an inverse association between low-density-lipoprotein cholesterol and mortality in the elderly: a systematic review. *BMJ Open.* 2016;6:e010401.

20. Kendrick M. *The great cholesterol con*. London: John Blake
    Publishing; 2008.
21. Scherstén T, Rosch PJ, Arfors KE, Sundberg R. The cholesterol hypoth-
    esis: time for the obituary? *Scand Cardiovasc J*. 2011;45(6):322–323.
22. Ravnskov U, DiNicolantonio JJ, Harcombe Z, et al. The questionable
    benefits of exchanging saturated fat with polyunsaturated fat. *Mayo
    Clin Proc*. 2014;89(4):451–453.
23. Hamazaki T, Okuyama H, Ogushi Y, Hama R. Cholesterol issues in
    Japan—why are the goals of cholesterol levels set so low? *Ann Nutr
    Metab*. 2013;62(1):32–36.
24. Sultan S, Hynes N. The ugly side of statins. Systematic appraisal of
    the contemporary un-known unknowns. *Open J Endocr Metab Dis*.
    2013;3(3):179–185.
25. Kendrick M. Cardiovascular disease is primarily due to blood clot-
    ting. In: Rosch PJ. *Fat and cholesterol don't cause heart attacks and statins
    are not the solution*. United Kingdom: Columbus Publishing; 2016.
26. Baroldi G, Silver MD. *The etiopathogenesis of coronary heart disease: a
    heretical theory based on morphology*. Boca Raton, FL: CRC Press; 2004.
27. Sroka K. Heart attack: new approaches. Various pages. http://
    heartattacknew.com/print-version/. Accessed March 15, 2017.
28. Sroka K. Acute blockage. http://heartattacknew.com/wp-content
    /uploads/2012/12/acute-blockage.pdf. Published December, 2012.
    Accessed March 15, 2017.
29. de Mesquita QH. Myogenic theory. Infarct Combat Project Web site.
    http://www.infarctcombat.org/MyogenicTheory.html. Accessed
    March 15, 2017.
30. Monteiro C. Infarct combat project. http://www.infarctcombat.org
    /cm/homepage.html. Accessed March 15, 2017.

Chapter Two: The Importance of Cholesterol

1. Krumholz H, Seeman TE, Merrill SS, et al. Lack of association
   between cholesterol and coronary heart disease mortality and
   morbidity and all-cause mortality in persons older than 70 years.
   JAMA. 1994;272(17):1335–1340.

2. Weverling-Rijnsburger AW, Blauw GJ, Lagaay AM, Knook DL, Meinders AE, Westendorp RG. Total cholesterol and risk of mortality in the oldest old. *Lancet.* 1997;350(9085):1119–1123.

3. Krum H, McMurray JJ. Statins and chronic heart failure: do we need a large-scale outcome trial? *J Am Coll Cardiol.* 2002; 39(10):1567–1573.

4. Böhm M, Hjalmarson A, Kjekshus J, et al. Heart failure and statins— why do we need a clinical trial? *ZS Kardiologie.* 2005;94(4):2223–2230.

5. Kjekshus J, Dunselman P, Blideskog M, et al. A statin in the treatment of heart failure? Controlled rosuvastatin multinational study in heart failure (CORONA): study design and baseline characteristics. *Eur J Heart Fail.* 2005;7(6):1059–1069.

6. Cleland JG, Loh H, Windram J, Goode K, Clark AL. Threats, opportunities, and statins in the modern management of heart failure. *Eur Heart J.* 2006;27(6):641–643.

7. Horwich TB, Hamilton MA, Maclellan WR, Fonarow GC. Low serum total cholesterol is associated with marked increase in mortality in advanced heart failure. *J Card Fail.* 2002;8(4):216–224.

8. Rauchhaus M, Clark AL, Doehner W, et al. The relationship between cholesterol and survival in patients with chronic heart failure. *J Am Coll Cardiol.* 2003;42(11):1933–1940.

9. Rauchhaus M, Coats AJ, Anker SD. The endotoxin-lipoprotein hypothesis. *Lancet.* 2000;356(9233):930–933.

10. Iribarren C, Jacobs Jr DR, Sidney S, Claxton AJ, Feingold KR. Cohort study of serum total cholesterol and in-hospital incidence of infectious diseases. *Epidemiol Infect.* 1998;121(2):335–347.

11. Schatz IJ, Masaki K, Yano K, Chen R, Rodriguez BL, Curb JD. Cholesterol and all-cause mortality in elderly people from the Honolulu Heart Program: a cohort study. *Lancet.* 2001;358(9279):351–355.

12. Huang X, Chen H, Miller WC, et al. Lower low-density lipoprotein cholesterol levels are associated with Parkinson's disease. *Mov Disord.* 2007;22(3):377–381.

13. Khot UN, Khot MB, Bajzer CT, et al. Prevalence of conventional risk factors in patients with coronary heart disease. *JAMA.* 2003;290(7):898–904.

14. Elias PK, Elias MF, D'Agostino RB, et al. Serum cholesterol and cognitive performance in the Framingham Heart Study. *Psychosom Med*. 2005;67(1):24–30.
15. Liu SY, Aliyari R, Li G, et al. Interferon-inducible cholesterol-25-hydroxylase broadly inhibits viral entry by production of 25-hydroxycholesterol. *Immunity*. 2013;38(1):92–105.
16. Cholesterol boosts the memory of the immune system. Science Daily. https://www.sciencedaily.com/releases/2012/12/121221081619.htm. Published December 21, 2012. Accessed June 7, 2017.
17. Sheng R, Chen Y, Gee HY, et al. Cholesterol modulates cell signaling and protein networking by specifically interacting with PDZ domain-containing scaffold proteins. *Nat Commun*. 2012;3:1249. doi:10.1038/ncomms2221
18. Theofilopoulos S, Wang Y, Kitambi SS, et al. Brain endogenous liver X receptor ligands selectively promote midbrain neurogenesis. *Nature Chem Biol*. 2013;9:126–133. doi:10.1038/nchembio.1156
19. Frost G, Leeds AA, Doré CJ, Madeiros S, Brading S, Dornhorst A. Glycaemic index as a determinant of serum HDL-cholesterol concentration. *Lancet*. 1999;353:1045–1048.
20. Foster GD, Wyatt HR, Hill JO, et al. A randomized trial of a low-carbohydrate diet for obesity. *N Engl J Med*. 2003;348(21):2082–2090.
21. Atkins, RC. *Dr. Atkins' new diet revolution*. New York: Avon Books; 1999.
22. Shai I, Schwarzfuchs D, Henkin Y, et al. Weight loss with a low-carbohydrate, Mediterranean, or low-fat diet. *N Engl J Med*. 2008;359(20):229–241.
23. Brehm BJ, Seeley RJ, Daniels SR, et al. A randomized trial comparing a very low carbohydrate diet and a calorie-restricted low fat diet on body weight and cardiovascular risk factors in healthy women. *The J Clin Endocrinol Metab*. 2003;88(4):1617–1623.
24. Stern L, Iqbal N, Seshadri P, et al. The effects of low-carbohydrate versus conventional weight loss diets in severely obese adults: one-year follow-up of a randomized trial. *Ann Intern Med*. 2004;140(10):778–785.

25. Yancy WS, Olsen MK, Guyton JR, Bakst RP, Westman EC. A low-carbohydrate, ketogenic diet versus a low-fat diet to treat obesity and hyperlipidemia. *Ann Intern Med.* 2004;140(10):769–777.

26. Gardner CD, Kiazand A, Alhassan S, et al. Comparison of the Atkins, Zone, Ornish and LEARN diets for change in weight and related risk factors among overweight premenopausal women. *JAMA.* 2007;297(2):969–977.

27. Liu S, Willett WC, Stampfer MJ, et al. A prospective study of dietary glycemic load, carbohydrate intake, and risk of coronary heart disease in US women. *Am J Clin Nutr.* 2000;71(6):1455–1461.

28. Mozaffarian D, Rimm EB, Herrington DM. Dietary fats, carbohydrate, and progression of coronary atherosclerosis in postmenopausal women. *Am J Clin Nutr.* 2004;80(5):1175–1184.

29. Ravnskov, U. The questionable role of saturated and polyunsaturated fatty acids in cardiovascular disease. *J Clin Epidemiol.* 1998; 51(6):443–460.

30. Siri-Tarino PW, Sun Q, Hu FB, Krauss RM. Meta-analysis of prospective cohort studies evaluating the association of saturated fat with cardiovascular disease. *Am J Clin Nutr.* 2010;91(3):535–546.

31. Kratz M, Baars T, Guyenet S. The relationship between high-fat dairy consumption and obesity, cardiovascular, and metabolic disease. *Eur J Nutr.* 2013;52(1):1–24.

32. Elwood PC, Pickering JE, Givens DI, Gallacher JE. The consumption of milk and dairy foods and the incidence of vascular disease and diabetes: an overview of the evidence. *Lipids.* 2010;45(10):925–939.

33. Barnes B, Barnes C. *Solved: the riddle of heart attacks.* Fort Collins, CO: Robinson Press; 1976.

34. Klein I, Danzi S. Thyroid disease and the heart. *Circulation.* 2007;116 (15):1725–1735 doi:10.1161/CIRCULATIONAHA.106.678326

35. Rizos CV, Elisaf MS, Liberopoulos EN. Effects of thyroid dysfunction on lipid profile. *Open Cardiovasc Med J.* 2011;5:76–84.

36. Jung, CH, Sung KC, Shin HS, et al. Thyroid dysfunction and their relation to cardiovascular risk factors such as lipid profile, hsCRP, and waist hip ratio in Korea. *Korean J Intern Med.* 2013;18(3):146–153.

Chapter Three: The Business of Selling Drugs

1. Office for National Statistics. Prescriptions dispensed in the community, England 2005–2015. July 5, 2016. http://content.digital.nhs.uk/catalogue/PUB20664/pres-disp-com-eng-2005-15-rep.pdf. Accessed March 7, 2017.

2. Smith R. *The trouble with medical journals*. Royal Society of Medicine Press Ltd., London, 2006.

3. Moynihan R, Heath I, Henry D. Selling sickness: the pharmaceutical industry and disease mongering. *BMJ*. 2002;324(7342):886–891.

4. Mintzes B. Disease mongering in drug promotion: do governments have a regulatory role? *PLoS Med*. 2006;3(4):0461–0465.

5. Heath I. Combating disease mongering: daunting but nonetheless essential. *PLoS Med*. 2006;3(4):0448–0451.

6. Primatesta P, Poulter NR. Lipid concentrations and the use of lipid lowering drugs: evidence from a national cross sectional survey. *BMJ*. 2000;321(7272):1322–1325.

7. Bruckert E. Epidemiology of low HDL-cholesterol: results of studies and surveys. *Eur Heart J*. 2006;8(Supplement F):F17–F22.

8. Associated Press. Cholesterol guidelines become a morality play. *USA Today*. October 16, 2004. http://usatoday30.usatoday.com/news/health/2004-10-16-panel-conflict-of-interest_x.htm. Accessed May 31, 2017.

9. Campbell EG, Gruen RL, Mountford J, Miller LG, Cleary PD, Blumenthal D. A national survey of physician-industry relationships. *N Eng J Med*. 2007;356(5):1742–1750.

10. Campbell EG. Doctors and drug companies—scrutinizing influential relationships. *N Eng J Med*. 2007;357(18):1796–1797.

11. Wazana A. Physicians and the pharmaceutical industry: is a gift ever just a gift? *JAMA*. 2000;283(3):373–380.

12. Lexchin J, Bero LA, Djulbegovic B, Clark O. Pharmaceutical industry sponsorship and research outcome and quality: systematic review. *BMJ*. 2003;326(7400):1167–1170.

13. Sterne JAC, Egger M, Smith GD. Investigating and dealing with publication and other biases in meta-analysis. *BMJ*. 2001;323(7304):101–105.

14. Berenson A. Study reveals doubt on drug for cholesterol. *New York Times*. January 18, 2008. http://www.nytimes.com/2008/01/15/business/15drug.html. Accessed March 9, 2017.
15. FierceBiotech. Merck/Schering-Plough Pharmaceuticals provides results of the ENHANCE trial. http://www.fiercebiotech.com/biotech/merck-schering-plough-pharmaceuticals-provides-results-of-enhance-trial. Published January 14, 2008. Accessed March 9, 2017.
16. Berenson A. Data about Zetia risks was not fully revealed. *New York Times*. December 21, 2007. http://www.nytimes.com/2007/12/21/business/21drug.html. Accessed March 9, 2017.
17. Bourne J. The NHS has spent £74 million on a new heart pill that the makers knew didn't work. How could this happen? *Daily Mail*. February 14, 2008.
18. Goldacre B. Clinical trials and playing by the rules. *Guardian*. January 5, 2008. https://www.theguardian.com/commentisfree/2008/jan/05/1. Accessed March 9, 2017.
19. Rossebø AB, Pedersen TR, Boman K, et al. Intensive lipid lowering with simvastatin and ezetimibe in aortic stenosis. *N Engl J Med*. 2008;359(13):1343–1356. doi:10.1056/NEJMoa0804602
20. Peto R, Emberson J, Landray M, et al. Analyses of cancer data from three ezetimibe trials. *N Engl J Med*. 2008;359(13):1357–1366. doi:10.1056/NEJMsa0806603
21. Drazen JM, D'Agostino RB, Ware JH, Morrissey S, Curfman GD. Ezetimibe and cancer—an uncertain association. *N Engl J Med*. 2008;359(13):1398–1399. doi:10.1056/NEJMe0807200
22. Berenson A. Cholesterol as a danger has skeptics. *New York Times*. January 17, 2008. Available at http://query.nytimes.com/gst/fullpage.html?res=9A01E0D6133FF934A25752C0A96E9C8B63. Accessed March 9, 2017.
23. Turner EH. Selective publication of antidepressant trials and its influence on apparent efficacy. *N Engl J Med*. 2008;358(3):252–260.
24. Kirsch I, Deacon BJ, Huedo-Medina TB, Scoboria A, Moore TJ, Johnson BT. Initial severity and antidepressant benefits: a meta-analysis

of data submitted to the Food and Drug Administration. *PLoS Med.* 2008;5(2):0260–0268.

25. Schwitzer G, Mudur G, Henry D, et al. What are the roles and responsibilities of the media in disseminating health information? *PLoS Med.* 2005;2(8):0576–0582.

26. British Heart Foundation. *Coronary heart disease statistics 2012.* London: British Heart Foundation; 2012.

27. Wager E. Authors, ghosts, damned lies, and statisticians. *PLoS Med.* 2007; 4(1):0005–0006.

28. Gøtzsche PC, Hróbjartsson A, Johansen HK, Haahr MT, Altman DG, Chan AW. Ghost authorship in industry-initiated randomised trials. *PLoS Med.* 2007;4(1):0047–0052.

Chapter Four: The Trouble with Statins

1. Hawkes N. The pill of life that keeps on working. *Times.* October 11, 2007.

2. Downs JR, Clearfield M, Weis S, et al. Primary prevention of acute coronary events with lovastatin in men and women with average cholesterol levels: results of AFCAPS/TexCAPS. *JAMA.* 1998;279(20):1615–1622.

3. Sever PS, Dahlöf B, Poulter NF, et al. Prevention of coronary and stroke events with atorvastatin in hypertensive patients who have average or lower-than-average cholesterol concentrations, in the Anglo-Scandinavian Cardiac Outcomes Trial—Lipid Lowering Arm (ASCOT-LLA): a multicentre randomised controlled trial. *Lancet.* 2003;361(9364):1149–1158.

4. Baigent C, Keech A, Kearney PM, et al. Efficacy and safety of cholesterol lowering treatment: prospective meta-analysis of data from 90,056 participants in 14 randomised trials of statins. *Lancet.* 2005;366(9493):1267–1278.

5. Cholesterol Treatment Trialists' (CTT) Collaborators, Kearney PM, Blackwell L, et al. Efficacy of cholesterol- lowering therapy in 18686 people with diabetes in 14 randomised trials of statins: a meta-analysis. *Lancet.* 2008;371(9607):117–125.

6. Heart Protection Study Collaborative Group. MRC/BHF Heart Protection Study of cholesterol lowering with simvastatin in 20,536 high-risk individuals: a randomised placebo-controlled trial. *Lancet*. 2002;360(9326):7–22.

7. Randomised trial of cholesterol lowering in 4444 patients with coronary heart disease: the Scandinavian Simvastatin Survival Study (4S). *Lancet*. 1994;344(8934):1383–1389.

8. Deedwania P, Barter P, Carmena R, et al. Reduction of low-density lipoprotein cholesterol in patients with coronary heart disease and metabolic syndrome: analysis of the Treating to New Targets study. *Lancet*. 2006;368(9539):919–928.

9. Shepherd J, Cobbe SM, Ford I, et al. Prevention of coronary heart disease with pravastatin in men with hypercholesterolemia. *N Eng J Med*. 1995;333(20):1301–1308.

10. British Heart Foundation. Statins page. https://www.bhf.org.uk /heart-health/treatments/statins. Accessed November 19, 2007.

11. Samani NJ, de Bono DP. Prevention of coronary heart disease with pravastatin. *N Eng J Med*. 1996;334(20):1333–1334; author reply 1334–1335.

12. British Heart Foundation. *Coronary heart disease statistics 2008*. London: British Heart Foundation; 2008.

13. Bakhru A, Erlinger TP. Smoking cessation and cardiovascular disease risk factors: results from the third National Health and Nutrition Examination Survey. *PloS Med*., 2005;v.2(6):0528–0536. doi:10.1371 /journal.pmed.0020160

14. Ford I, Murray H, Packard CJ, et al. Long-term follow-up of the west of Scotland coronary prevention study. *N Eng J Med*. 2007;357(15): 1477–1486.

15. Domanski MJ. Primary prevention of coronary artery disease. *N Eng J Med*. 2007;357(15):1543–1545.

16. Ray KK, Seshasai SR, Erqou S, et al. Statins and all-cause mortality in high-risk primary prevention: a meta-analysis of 11 randomized controlled trials involving 65,229 participants. *Arch Intern Med*. 2010;170(12):1024–1031.

17. Hughes S. Cochrane review stirs controversy over statins in primary prevention. TheHeart.org. January 20, 2011. http://www.medscape.com/viewarticle/736131. Accessed March 15, 2017.

18. The NNT. http://www.thennt.com/nnt/statins-for-heart-disease-prevention-without-prior-heart-disease. Accessed March 4, 2017.

19. Zacharski LR, DePalma RG, Shamayeva G, Chow BK. The statin-iron nexus: anti-inflammatory intervention for arterial disease prevention. *Am J Public Health*. 2013;103(4)e105–e112 epub ahead of print. Accessed March 15, 2017.

20. Okuyama H, Langsjoen PH, Hamazaki T, et al. Statins stimulate atherosclerosis and heart failure: pharmacological mechanisms. *Expert Rev Clin Pharmacol*. 2015;8(2):189–199.

21. Hamazaki T, Okuyama H, Ogushi Y, Hama R. Towards a paradigm shift in cholesterol treatment. a re-examination of the cholesterol issue in japan. *Ann Nutr Metab*. 2015;66(suppl 4):1–116.

22. Kristensen ML, Christensen PM, Hallas J. The effect of statins on average survival in randomised trials, an analysis of end point postponement. *BMJ Open*. 2015;5:e007118. doi:10.1136/bmjopen-2014-007118

23. Mortensen SA, Leth A, Agner E, Rohde M. Dose-related decrease of serum coenzyme q10 during treatment with HMG-CoA reductase inhibitors. *Mol Aspects Med*. 1997;18 Suppl:S137–S144.

24. Borel P, Moussa M, Reboul E, et al. Human plasma levels of vitamin E and carotenoids are associated with genetic polymorphisms in genes involved in lipid metabolism. *J Nutr*. 2007;137(12):2653–2659.

25. Packer L, Fuchs J, eds. *Vitamin E in health and disease*. New York: CRC Press; 1992.

26. Benowicz RJ. *Vitamins and you: a simple no-nonsense guide to the intelligent use of natural and synthetic vitamins*. New York: Grosset and Dunlap; 1979.

27. DeCava JA. *The real truth about vitamins and anti-oxidants*, 2nd edition. Fort Collins, CO: Selene River Press; 2006.

28. Colpo A. *The great cholesterol con: why everything you've been told about cholesterol, diet and heart disease is wrong!* LULU; 2006.

29. Barter PJ, Caulfield M, Eriksson M, et al. Effects of torcetrapib in patients at high risk for coronary events. *N Eng J Med*. 2007;357(21):2109–2122.

30. Psaty BM, Furberg CD, Ray WA, et al. Potential for conflict of interest in the evaluation of suspected adverse drug reactions: use of cerivastatin and risk of rhabdomyolysis. *JAMA*. 2004;292(21):2622–2631.

31. Weber W. Drug firm withdraws statin from the market. *Lancet*. 2001;358(9281):568.

32. Lee K, Bacchetti P, Sim I. Publication of clinical trials supporting successful new drug applications: a literature analysis. *PLoS Med*. 2008;5(9):e191. doi:10.1371/journal.pmed.0050191

33. Ravnskov U, Rosch PJ, Sutter MC, Houston MC. Should we lower cholesterol as much as possible? *BMJ*. 2006;332:1330–1332.

34. Kendrick M. Should women be offered cholesterol lowering drugs to prevent cardiovascular disease? No. *BMJ*. 2007;334(7601):983.

35. Gale EA. Lessons from the glitazones: a story of drug development. *Lancet*. 2001;357(9271):1870–1875.

36. Shepherd J, Blauw GJ, Murphy MB, et al. Pravastatin in elderly individuals at risk of vascular disease (PROSPER): a randomised controlled trial. *Lancet*. 2002;360(9346):1623–1630.

37. Ravnskov U, McCully KS, Rosch PJ. The statin-low cholesterol-cancer conundrum. *QJM*. 2012;105(4):383–388.

38. Graveline D. *Lipitor, thief of memory: statin drugs and the misguided war on cholesterol*. Amazon Digital Services LLC; 2010.

39. Wagstaff LR, Mitton MW, Arvik BM, Doraiswamy PM. Statin-associated memory loss: analysis of 60 case reports and review of the literature. *Pharmacotherapy*. 2003;23(7):871–880.

40. King DS, Wilburn AJ, Wofford MR, Harrell TK, Lindley BJ, Jones DW. Cognitive impairment associated with atorvastatin and simvastatin. *Pharmacotherapy*. 2003;23(12):1663–1667.

41. Golomb BA, Kane T, Dimsdale JE. Severe irritability associated with statin cholesterol lowering. *QJM*. 2004;97(4):229–235.

42. Kraft R, Kahn A, Medina-Franco J, et al. A cell-based fascin bioassay identifies compounds with potential anti-metastasis or cognition-enhancing functions. *Dis Model Mech*. 2012;6(1):217–235.

43. Rizvi K, Hampson JP, Harvey JN. Do lipid-lowering drugs cause erectile dysfunction? A systematic review. *Fam Pract.* 2002;19(1):95–98.

44. de Graaf L, Brouwers AH, Diemont WL. Is decreased libido associated with the use of HMG-CoA-reductase inhibitors? *Br J Clin Pharmacol.* 2004;58(3):326–328.

45. Tomlinson SS, Mangione KK. Potential adverse effects of statins on muscle. *Phys Ther.* 2005;85(5):459–465.

46. Edison RJ, Muenke M. Central nervous system and limb anomalies in case reports of first-trimester statin exposure. *N Eng J Med.* 2004;350(15):1579.

47. Pasternak RC, Smith SC, Bairey-Merz CN, Grundy SM, Cleeman JI, Lenfant C. ACC/AHA/NHLBI clinical advisory on the use and safety of statins. *Circulation.* 2002;106(8):1024–1028.

48. Ucar M, Mjorndal T, Dahlqvist R. HMG-CoA reductase inhibitors and myotoxicity. *Drug Saf.* 2000;22(6):441–457.

49. Cannon CP, Braunwald E, McCabe CH, et al. Intensive versus moderate lipid lowering with statins after acute coronary syndromes. *N Eng J Med.* 2004;350(15):1495–1504.

50. Sinzinger H, Wolfram R, Peskar BA. Muscular side effects of statins. *J Cardiovasc Pharmacol.* 2002;40(2):163–171.

51. Wise SJ, Nathoo NA, Etminan M, Mikelberg FS, Mancini GB. Statin use and risk for cataract: A nested case-control study of 2 populations in Canada and the United States. *Can J Cardiol.* 2014;30(12):1613–1619.

52. Nakazato R, Gransar H, Berman DS, et al. Statins use and coronary artery plaque composition: Results from the International Multicenter Confirm Registry. *Atherosclerosis.* 2012;225(1):148–153.

53. Raggi P, Davidson M, Callister TQ, et al.. Aggressive versus moderate lipid-lowering therapy in hypercholesterolemic postmenopausal women: beyond endorsed lipid lowering with EBT scanning (BELLES). *Circulation.* 2005;112(4):563–571. doi:10.1161/CIRCULATIONAHA.104.512681

54. Schmermund A, Achenbach S, Budde T, et al. Effect of intensive versus standard lipid-lowering treatment with atorvastatin on the progression of calcified coronary atherosclerosis over 12

months: a multicenter, randomized, double-blind trial. *Circulation.*
2006;113(3):427–437. doi:10.1161/CIRCULATIONAHA.105.568147

55. Saremi R, Bahn G, Reaven PD, et al. Progression of vascular calcification is increased with statin use in the Veterans Affairs Diabetes
Trial (VADT). *Diabetes Care.* 2012;35(11).2390–2392. doi:10.2337
/dc12-0464

56. Mikus CR, Boyle LJ, Borengasser SJ, et al. Simvastatin impairs
exercise training adaptations. *J Am Coll Cardiol.* 2013;62(8):709–714.

Chapter Five: The Real Causes of Heart Disease

1. American Heart Association. Managing stress to control high blood
pressure page. http://www.heart.org/HEARTORG/Conditions
/HighBloodPressure/PreventionTreatmentofHighBloodPressure
/Stress-and-Blood-Pressure_UCM_301883_Article.jsp#.V7
_7s8ekz8N. Accessed August 25, 2016.

2. Smith J. *Statin nation: the great cholesterol cover-up* [DVD]. 2012.

3. Smith J. *Statin nation II: what really causes heart disease* [DVD]. 2015.

4. Scarborough P, Bhatnagar P, Wickramasinghe K, Smolina K, Mitchell
C, Rayner M. *Coronary heart disease statistics 2010 edition.* British
Heart Foundation Health Promotion Research Group, Department
of Public Health, University of Oxford; 2010.

5. Allender S, Peto V, Scarborough P, Kaur A, Rayner M. *Coronary
heart disease statistics 2008 edition.* British Heart Foundation Health
Promotion Research Group, Department of Public Health, University of Oxford; 2008.

6. Ferrie JE, ed. Work stress and health: the Whitehall II study. London:
Public and Commercial Services Union on behalf of Council of
Civil Service Unions/Cabinet Office; 2004. https://www.ucl.ac.uk
/whitehallII/pdf/wii-booklet. Accessed August 25, 2016.

7. Björntorp P, Rosmond R. Obesity and cortisol. *Nutrition.*
2000;16(10):924–936.

8. Airaksinen KE, Ikäheimo MJ, Linnaluoto MK, Niemelä M, Takku-
nen JT. Impaired vagal heart rate control in coronary heart disease.
Br Heart J. 1987;58(6):592–597.

9. Bigger JT, Fleiss JL, Steinman RC, Rolnitzky LM, Schneider WJ, Stein PK. RR variability in healthy, middle-aged persons compared with patients with chronic coronary heart disease or recent acute myocardial infarction. *Circulation*. 1995;91(7):1936–1943.

10. Burger AJ, Hamer AW, Weinrauch LA, D'elia JA. Relation of heart rate variability and serum lipoproteins in type 1 diabetes mellitus and chronic stable angina pectoris. *Am J Cardiol*. 1998; 81(8):945–949.

11. Burger AJ, Kamalesh M. Effect of beta-adrenergic blocker therapy on the circadian rhythm of heart rate variability in patients with chronic stable angina pectoris. *Am J Cardiol*. 1999; 83(4):596–598.

12. Hayano J, Sakakibara Y, Yamada M, et al. Decreased magnitude of heart rate spectral components in coronary artery disease. Its relation to angiographic severity. *Circulation*. 1990;81(4):1217–1224. doi:10.1161/01.CIR.81.4.1217

13. Hayano J, Yamada A, Mukai S, et al. Severity of coronary atherosclerosis correlates with the respiratory component of heart rate variability. *Am Heart J*. 1991;121(4 Pt 1):1070–1079.

14. Liao D, Cai J, Rosamond WD, et al. Cardiac autonomic function and incident coronary heart disease: a population-based case-cohort study. The ARIC Study. *Am J Epidemiol*. 1997;145(8):696–706.

15. Mäkikallio TH, Ristimäe T, Airaksinen KE, Peng CK, Goldberger AL, Huikuri HV. Heart rate dynamics in patients with stable angina pectoris and utility of fractal and complexity measures. *Am J Cardiol*. 1998;81(1):27–31.

16. Nolan J, Flapan AD, Goodfield NE, et al. Measurement of parasympathetic activity from 24-hour ambulatory electrocardiograms and its reproducibility and sensitivity in normal subjects, patients with symptomatic myocardial ischemia, and patients with diabetes mellitus. *Am J Cardiol*. 1996;77(2):154–158.

17. Tsuji H, Larson MG, Venditti FJ, et al. Impact of reduced heart rate variability on risk for cardiac events. The Framingham Heart Study. *Circulation*. 1996;94(11):2850–2855.

18. Wennerblom B, Lurje L, Solem J, et al. Reduced heart rate variability in ischemic heart disease is only partially caused by ischemia. *Cardiology*. 2000;94(3):146–151.

19. Nolan J, Flapan AD, Reid J, Neilson JM, Bloomfield P, Ewing DJ. Cardiac parasympathetic activity in severe uncomplicated coronary artery disease. *Br Heart J*. 1994;71(6):515–520.

20. Rich MW, Saini JS, Kleiger RE, Carney RM, teVelde A, Freedland KE. Correlation of heart rate variability with clinical and angiographic variables and late mortality after coronary angiography. *Am J Cardiol*. 1988;62(10 Pt 1):714–717.

21. Takase B, Kurita A, Noritake M, et al. Heart rate variability in patients with diabetes mellitus, ischemic heart disease, and congestive heart failure. *J Electrocardiol*. 1992;25(2):79–88.

22. Dekker JM, Schouten EG, Klootwijk P, Pool J, Swenne CA, Kromhout D. Heart rate variability from short electrocardiographic recordings predicts mortality from all causes in middle-aged and elderly men: the Zutphen study. *Am J Epidemiol*. 1997;145(10):899–908.

23. Huikuri HV, Mäkikallio TH, Airaksinen KE, et al. Power-law relationship of heart rate variability as a predictor of mortality in the elderly. *Circulation*. 1998;97(20):2031–2036.

24. Mäkikallio TH, Huikuri HV, Mäkikallio A, et al. Prediction of sudden cardiac death by fractal analysis of heart rate variability in elderly subjects. *J Am Coll Cardiol*. 2001;37(5):1395–1402.

25. Mäkikallio TH, Høiber S, Køber L, et al. Fractal analysis of heart rate dynamics as a predictor of mortality in patients with depressed left ventricular function after acute myocardial infarction. *Am J Cardiol*. 1999;83(6):836–839.

26. Huikuri HV, Mäkikallio TH, Chung-Kang P, et al. Fractal correlation properties of R-R interval dynamics and mortality in patients with depressed left ventricular function after an acute myocardial infarction. *Circulation*. 2000;101(1):47–53.

27. Kop WJ, Verdino RJ, Gottdiener JS, O'Leary ST, Bairey Merz CN, Krantz DS. Changes in heart rate and heart rate variability before ambulatory ischemic events. *J Am Coll Cardiol*. 2001;38(3):742–749.

28. Tuininga YS, Crijns HJ, Brouwer J, et al. Evaluation of importance of central effects of atenolol and metoprolol measured by heart rate variability during mental performance tasks, physical exercise, and daily life in stable postinfarct patients. *Circulation.* 1995;92(12):3415–3423.

29. Sroka K. On the genesis of myocardial ischemia. *Z Kardiol.* 2004;93(10):768–783.

30. Scheuer J. Myocardial metabolism in cardiac hypoxia. *Am J Cardiol.* 1967;19(3):385–392.

31. Monteiro C. *Acidity theory of atherosclerosis: new evidences.* CreateSpace; 2012.

32. Katz AM. Effects of ischemia on the cardiac contractile proteins. *Cardiology.* 1971;56(1):276–283.

33. Monteiro CE. Stress as cause of atherosclerosis: the acidity theory. In: Rosch J, ed. *Fat and cholesterol don't cause heart attacks and statins are not the solution.* Columbus Publishing; 2016.

34. Kendrick M. Cardiovascular disease is primarily due to blood clotting. In: Rosch J, ed. *Fat and cholesterol don't cause heart attacks and statins are not the solution.* Columbus Publishing; 2016.

35. Opie LH. Acute metabolic response in myocardial infarction. *Br Heart J.* 1971;33Suppl:129–137.

36. Katz LN, Long CN. Lactic acid in mammalian cardiac muscle. Part 1. The stimulation maximum. Proceedings of the Royal Society. Series B. *Biol Sci.*1925;99:8.

37. Tennant R. Factors concerning the arrest of contraction in an ischemic myocardial area. *Am J Physiol.* 1935;113:677–682.

38. Schneider RH, Grim CE, Rainforth MV, et al. Stress reduction in the secondary prevention of cardiovascular disease: randomized, controlled trial of transcendental meditation and health education in blacks. *Circ Cardiovasc Qual Outcomes.* 2012;5(6):750–758. doi:10.1161/CIRCOUTCOMES.112.967406.

39. Smith J. *$29 billion reasons to lie about cholesterol.* Troubador: 2009.

40. Randomised trial of cholesterol lowering in 4444 patients with coronary heart disease: the Scandinavian Simvastatin Survival Study (4S). *Lancet.* 1994;344(8934):1383–1389.

41. Kwon HM, Sangiogi G, Ritman EL, et al. Enhanced coronary vasa vasorum neovascularization in experimental hypercholesterolemia. *J Clin Invest*. 1998;101(8):1551–1556.

42. Ravnskov U. Uffe Ravnskov homepage. http://www.ravnskov.nu. Accessed March 15, 2017.

43. Ravnskov U. *The cholesterol myths*. White Plains, MD: NewTrends Publishing; 2000.

44. Ravnskov U, McCully K. Vulnerable plaque formation from obstruction of vasa vasorum by homocysteinylated and oxidized lipoprotein aggregates complexed with microbial remnants and LDL autoantibodies. *Ann Clin Lab Sci*. 2009;39(1):3–16.

45. Thayer WS. On the cardiac and vascular complications and sequels of typhoid fever. *Bull Johns Hopkins Hosp*. 1904;Oct:323–340.

46. Wiesel J. Die erkrankungen arterieller gefässe im verlaufe akuter infektionen. II Teil. *Z Heilkunde*. 1906;27:262–294.

47. Madjid M, Miller CC, Zarubaev VV, et al. Influenza epidemics and acute respiratory disease activity are associated with a surge in autopsy-confirmed coronary heart disease death: results from 8 years of autopsies in 34,892 subjects. *Eur Heart J*. 2007;28(10): 1205–1210.

48. Smeeth L, Thomas SL, Hall AJ, Hubbard R, Farrington P, Vallance P. Risk of myocardial infarction and stroke after acute infection or vaccination. *N Eng J Med*. 2004;351(25):2611–2618.

49. Valtonen V, Kuikka A, Syrjänen J. Thromboembolic complications in bacteremic infections. *Eur Heart J*. 1993;14SupplK:20–23.

50. Spahr A, Klein E, Khuseyinova N, et al. Periodontal infections and coronary heart disease: role of periodontal bacteria and importance of total pathogen burden in the Coronary Event and Periodontal Disease (CORODONT) study. *Arch Intern Med*. 2006;166(5):554–549.

51. Khamis RY, Hughes AD, Caga-Anan M, et al. high serum immunoglobulin g and m levels predict freedom from adverse cardiovascular events in hypertension: a nested case-control substudy of the Anglo-Scandinavian Cardiac Outcomes Trial. *EBioMedicine*. 2016;9:372–380.

52. Immune system linked to lower heart attack risk, suggests study. *Science Daily*. June 20, 2016. https://www.sciencedaily.com/releases/2016/06/160620085208.htm. Accessed March 15, 2017.

53. He J, Vupputuri S, Allen K, Prerost MR, Hughes J, Whelton PK. Passive smoking and the risk of coronary heart disease—a meta-analysis of epidemiologic studies. *N Eng J Med*. 1999;340(12):920–926.

54. Glantz SA, Parmley WW. Passive smoking and heart disease. Mechanisms and risk. *JAMA*. 1995;273:1047–1053.

55. Dockery DW. Health effects of particulate air pollution. *Ann Epidemiol*. 2009;19(4):257–263.

56. Bhatnagar A. Environmental cardiology: studying mechanistic links between pollution and heart disease. *Circ Res*. 2006;99(7):692–705.

57. Pope CA 3rd, Burnett RT, Thurston GD, et al. Cardiovascular mortality and long-term exposure to particulate air pollution: epidemiological evidence of general pathophysiological pathways of disease. *Circulation*. 2004;109(1):71–77.

58. Dominici F, Peng RD, Bell ML, et al. Fine particulate air pollution and hospital admission for cardiovascular and respiratory diseases. *JAMA*. 2006;295(10):1127–1134.

59. Peters A, Dockery DW, Muller JE, Mittleman MA. Increased particulate air pollution and the triggering of myocardial infarction. *Circulation*. 2001;103(23):2810–2815.

60. Miller KA, Siscovick DS, Sheppard L, et al. Long-term exposure to air pollution and incidence of cardiovascular events in women. *NEJM*. 2007; 356(5):447–458.

61. Gold DR, Litonjua A, Schwartz J, et al. Ambient pollution and heart rate variability. *Circulation*. 2000;101(11):1267–1273.

62. Magari SR, Hauser R, Schwartz J, Williams PL, Smith TJ, Christiani DC. Association of heart rate variability with occupational and environmental exposure to particulate air pollution. *Circulation*. 2001;104(9):986–991.

63. Pope CA 3rd, Verrier RL, Lovett EG, et al. Heart rate variability associated with particulate air pollution. *Am Heart J*. 1999;138 (5 Pt 1):890–899.

64. Riediker M, Cascio WE, Griggs TR, et al. Particulate matter exposure in cars is associated with cardiovascular effects in healthy young men. *Am J Respir Crit Care Med.* 2004;169(8):934–940.

65. World Health Organization. Public health, environmental and social determinants of health (PHE). WHO Global Urban Ambient Air Pollution Database (update 2016). http://www.who.int/phe/health _topics/outdoorair/databases/cities/en. Accessed March 15, 2017.

66. Liboff AR. Medical problems arising from solar storms. In: Rosch PJ, ed. *Bioelectromagnetic and subtle energy medicine, 2nd edition.* Boca Raton, FL: CRC Press; 2015.

67. Sun spots affect some maladies French doctors believe they have proved. *New York Times,* July 12, 1922:1.

68. Halberg F, Düll-Pfaff N, Gumarova L, et al. 27-day cycles in human mortality: Traute and Bernhard Düll. *Hist Geo Space Sci.* 2013;4. doi:10.5194/hgss-4-47-2013

69. Vencluviene J, Babarskiene R, Slapikas R, Sakalyte G. The association between phenomena on the sun, geomagnetic activity, meteorological variables, and cardiovascular characteristic in patients with myocardial infarction. *Int J Biometeor,* 2013;57(5):797–804.

70. Mendoza B, Diaz-Sandoval R. Relationship between solar activity and myocardial infarctions in Mexico City. *Geofis Int.* 2000;39(1):53–56.

71. Rodriguez-Tabbada RE, Figueredo PS, Figueredo SS. Geomagnetic activity related to acute myocardial infarctions: Relationship in a reduced population and time interval. *Geofis Int.* 2004;43(2):265–269.

72. Stoupel E, Kalediene R, Petrauskiene J, et al. Twenty years study of solar, geomagnetic, cosmic ray activity links with monthly deaths numbers (n-850304). *J Biomed Sci Eng.* 2011;4(6):426–434.

73. Cornéllisen G, Halberg F, Breus T, et al. Non-photic solar associations of heart rate variability and myocardial infarction. *J Atm Solar Terr Phys.* 2002;64(5-6):707–720.

74. Cornelissen G, Watanabe Y, Otsuka K, Halberg F. Influences of space and terrestrial weather on human physiology and pathology. In: Rosch PJ, ed. *Bioelectromagnetic and subtle energy medicine, 2nd edition.* Boca Raton, FL: CRC Press; 2015.

Chapter Six: CoQ10 and the Heart's Energy Factory

1. Murray AJ, Edwards LM, Clarke K. Mitochondria and heart failure. *Curr Opin Clin Nutr Metab Care.* 2007;10(6):704–711.
2. Chen L, Knowlton AA. Mitochondrial dynamics in heart failure. *Congest Heart Fail.* 2011;17(6):257–261.
3. Alehagen U, Johansson P, Björnstedt M, Rosén A, Dahlström U. Cardiovascular mortality and N-terminal proBNP reduced after combined selenium and CoQ10 supplementation: a 5-year prospective randomized double-blind placebo-controlled trial among elderly Swedish citizens. *Int J Cardiol.* 2013;167(5):1860–1866.
4. Downs JR, Clearfield M, Weis S, et al. Primary prevention of acute coronary events with lovastatin in men and women with average cholesterol levels: results of AFCAPS/TexCAPS. *JAMA.* 1998;279(20):1615–1622.
5. Smith J. *Statin nation: the great cholesterol cover-up* [DVD]. 2012.
6. Lockwood K, Moesgaard S, Folkers K. Partial and complete regression of breast cancer in patients in relation to dosage of coenzyme Q10. *Biochem Biophys Res Commun.* 1994;199(3):1504–1508.
7. Rusciani L, Proietti I, Paradisi A, et al. Recombinant interferon alpha-2b and coenzyme Q10 as a postsurgical adjuvant therapy for melanoma: a 3-year trial with recombinant interferon-alpha and 5-year follow-up. *Melanoma Res.* 2007;17(3):177–183.
8. Okuyama H, Langsjoen PH, Hamazaki T, et al. Statins stimulate atherosclerosis and heart failure: pharmacological mechanisms. *Expert Rev Clin Pharmacol.* 2015;8(2):189–199.
9. Rayman MP. Selenium and human health. *Lancet.* 2012;379(9822): 1256–1268.
10. Flores-Mateo G, Navas-Acien A, Pastor-Barriuso R, Guallar E. Selenium and coronary heart disease: a meta-analysis. *Am J Clin Nutr.* 2006;84(4):762–773.
11. Bruce A. Swedish views on selenium. *Ann Clin Res.* 1986;18(1):8–12.
12. Alehagen U, Johannson P, Björnstedt M, Rosén A, Post C, Aaseth J. Relatively high mortality risk in elderly Swedish subjects with low selenium status. *Eur J Clin Nutr.* 2016;70(1):91–96.

13. Langsjoen PH, Langsjoen PH, Folkers K. A six year clinical study of therapy of cardiomyopathy with coenzyme Q10. *Int J Tissue React.* 1990;12(3):169–171.

14. Langsjoen PH, Langsjoen AM. Overview of the use of CoQ10 in cardiovascular disease. *Biofactors.* 1999;9(2-4):273–284.

15. Langsjoen PH, Langsjoen AM. Supplemental ubiquinol in patients with advanced congestive heart failure. *Biofactors.* 2008;32(1-4):119–128.

16. Morisco C, Trimarco B, Condorelli M. Effect of coenzyme Q10 therapy in patients with congestive heart failure: a long term multicenter randomized study. *Clin Invest.* 1993;71(8Suppl):134–136.

17. Soja AM, Mortensen SA. Treatment of congestive heart failure with coenzyme Q10 illuminated by meta-analyses of clinical trials. *Mol Aspects Med.*1997;18(Suppl):S159–168.

18. Sander S, Coleman CI, Patel AA, Kluger J, White CM. The impact of coenzyme Q10 on systolic function in patients with chronic heart failure. *J Card Fail.* 2006;12(6):464–472.

19. Fotino AD, Thompson-Paul AM, Bazzano L. Effect of coenzyme Q10 supplementation on heart failure: a meta-analysis. *Am J Clin Nutr.* 2013;97(2):268–275.

20. Mortensen SA, Rosenfeldt F, Kumar A, et al. The effect of coenzyme Q10 on morbidity and mortality in chronic heart failure. *JACC Heart Fail.* 2014;2(6):641–649.

21. British Heart Foundation. Treatments: drugs, stents and surgery. https://www.bhf.org.uk/research/what-we-research/treatments -drugs-stents-and-surgery. Accessed March 15, 2017.

22. Alberts B, Johnson A, Lewis J, et al. *Molecular biology of the cell. 4th edition.* New York: Garland Science; 2002.

23. Gao L, Mao Q, Cao J, Wang Y, Zhou X, Fan L. Effects of coenzyme Q10 on vascular endothelial function in humans: a meta-analysis of randomized controlled trials. *Atherosclerosis.* 2012;221(2):311–316.

24. Singh RB, Niaz MA, Rastogi SS, Shukla PK, Thakur AS. Effect of hydrosoluble COQ10 on blood pressure and insulin resistance in hypertensive patients with coronary artery disease. *J Hum Hypertens.* 1999;13(3):203–208.

25. Burke BE, Neuenschwander R, Olson RD. Randomized double-blind placebo controlled trial of coenzyme Q10 in isolated systolic hypertension. *South Med J.* 2001;94(11):1112–1117.

26. Rosenfeldt FL, Haas SJ, Krum H, et al. Coenzyme Q10 in the treatment of hypertension: a meta-analysis of clinical trials. *J Hum Hypertens.* 2007;21(4):297–306.

27. Lobo V, Patil A, Phatak A, Chandra N. Free radicals, antioxidants and functional foods: impact on human health. *Pharmacogn Rev.* 2010;4(8):118–126.

28. Shults CW, Flint Beal M, Song D, Fontaine D. Pilot trial of high dosages of coenzyme Q10 in patients with Parkinson's disease. *Exp Neurol.* 2004;188(2):491–494.

29. Ferrante KL, Shefner J, Zhang H, et al. Tolerance of high-dose (3000mg/day) coenzyme Q10 in ALS. *Neurology.* 2005;65(11):1834–1836.

Chapter Seven: Nutrition for the Heart

1. Foster GD, Wyatt HR, Hill JO, et al. A randomized trial of a low-carbohydrate diet for obesity. *N Eng J Med.* 2003;348(21):2082–2090.

2. Shai I, Schwarzfuchs D, Henkin Y, et al. Weight loss with a low-carbohydrate, Mediterranean, or low-fat diet. *N Eng J Med.* 2008;359(3):229–241.

3. Brehm BJ, Seeley RJ, Daniels SR, et al. A randomized trial comparing a very low carbohydrate diet and a calorie-restricted low fat diet on body weight and cardiovascular risk factors in healthy women. *J Clin Endocrinol Metabol.* 2003;88(4):1617–1623.

4. Stern L, Iqbal N, Seshadri P, et al. The effects of low-carbohydrate versus conventional weight loss diets in severely obese adults: one-year follow-up of a randomized trial. *Ann Intern Med.* 2004;140(10):778–785.

5. Yancy WS, Olsen MK, Guyton JR, Bakst RP, Westman EC. A low-carbohydrate, ketogenic diet versus a low-fat diet to treat obesity and hyperlipidemia. *Ann Intern Med.* 2004;140(10):769–777.

6. Gardner CD, Kiazand A, Alhassan S, et al. Comparison of the Atkins, Zone, Ornish and LEARN diets for change in weight and related risk factors among overweight premenopausal women. *JAMA.* 2007;297(9):969–977.

7. Liu S, Manson JE, Stampfer MJ, et al. Dietary glycemic load assessed by food-frequency questionnaire in relation to plasma high-density-lipoprotein cholesterol and fasting plasma triacylglycerols in postmenopausal women. *Am J Clin Nutr*. 2001;73(3):560–566.

8. Radhika G, Ganesan A, Sathya RM, Sudha V, Mohan V. Dietary carbohydrates, glycemic load and serum high-density lipoprotein cholesterol concentrations among south Indian adults. *Eur J Clin Nutr*. 2007;63(3):413–420.

9. Garg A, Grundy SM, Koffler M. Effect of high carbohydrate intake on hyperglycemia, islet function, and plasma lipoproteins in NIDDM. *Diabetes Care*. 1992;15(11):1572–1580.

10. Garg A, Bantle JP, Henry RR, et al. Effects of varying carbohydrate content of diet in patients with non-insulin-dependent diabetes mellitus. *JAMA*. 1994;271(18):1421–1428.

11. Samaha FF, Iqbal N, Seshadri P, et al. A low-carbohydrate as compared with a low-fat diet in severe obesity. *N Eng J Med*. 2003;348(21): 2074–2081.

12. Appel LJ, Sacks FM, Carey VJ, et al. Effects of protein, monounsaturated fat, and carbohydrate intake on blood pressure and serum lipids. *JAMA*. 2005;294(19):2455–2464.

13. Mozaffarian D, Rimm EB, Herrington DM. Dietary fats, carbohydrate, and progression of coronary atherosclerosis in postmenopausal women. *Am J Clin Nutr*. 2004;80(5):1175–1184.

14. Dunder K, Lind L, Zethelius B, Berglund L, Lithell H. Increase in blood glucose concentration during antihypertensive treatment as a predictor of myocardial infarction: population based cohort study. *BMJ*. 2003;326(7391):681–685.

15. Saydah SH, Miret M, Sung J, Varas C, Gause D, Brancati FL. Postchallenge hyperglycemia and mortality in a national sample of U.S. adults. *Diabetes Care*. 2001;24(8):1397–1402.

16. Qiao Q, Dekker JM, de Vegt F, et al. Two prospective studies found that elevated 2-hr glucose predicted male mortality independent of fasting glucose and HbA1c. *J Clin Epidemiol*. 2004;57(6):590–596.

17. Temelkova-Kurktschiev TS, Koehler C, Henkel E, Leonhardt W, Fuecker K, Hanefeld M. Postchallenge plasma glucose and glycemic spikes are more strongly associated with atherosclerosis than fasting glucose or HbA1c level. *Diabetes Care.* 2000;23(12):1830–1834.

18. Balkau B, Shipley M, Jarrett RJ, et al. High blood glucose concentration is a risk factor for mortality in middle-aged non-diabetic men. 20-year follow-up in the Whitehall Study, the Paris Prospective Study, and the Helsinki Policemen Study. *Diabetes Care.* 1998;21(3):360–367.

19. Liu S, Willett WC, Stampfer MJ, et al. A prospective study of dietary glycemic load, carbohydrate intake, and risk of coronary heart disease in US women. *Am J Clin Nutr.* 2000;71(6):1455–1461.

20. Levitan EB, Song Y, Ford ES, Liu S. Is nondiabetic hyperglycemia a risk factor for cardiovascular disease? A meta-analysis of prospective studies. *Arch Intern Med.* 2004;164(19):2147–2155.

21. Danaei G, Lawes CM, Vander Hoorn S, Murray CJ, Ezzati M. Global and regional mortality from ischaemic heart disease and stroke attributable to higher-than-optimum blood glucose concentration: comparative risk assessment. *Lancet.* 2006;368(9548): 1651–1659.

22. Wei M, Gaskill SP, Haffner SM, Stern MP. Effects of diabetes and level of glycemia on all-cause and cardiovascular mortality. The San Antonio Heart Study. *Diabetes Care.* 1998;21(7):1167–1172.

23. Rodriguez BL, Lau N, Burchfield CM, et al. Glucose intolerance and 23-year risk of coronary heart disease and total mortality: the Honolulu Heart Program. *Diabetes Care.* 1999;22(8):1262–1265.

24. Vaccaro O, Ruth KJ, Stamler J. Relationship of postload plasma glucose to mortality with 19-yr follow-up. Comparison of one versus two plasma glucose measurements in the Chicago Peoples Gas Company Study. *Diabetes Care.* 1992;15(10):1328–1334.

25. Lowe LP, Liu K, Greenland P, Metzger BE, Dyer AR, Stamler J. Diabetes, asymptomatic hyperglycemia, and 22-year mortality in black and white men. The Chicago Heart Association Detection Project in Industry Study. *Diabetes Care.* 1997;20(2):163–169.

26. Li Z, Otvos JD, Lamon-Fava S, et al. Men and women differ in lipo-protein response to dietary saturated fat and cholesterol restriction. *J Nutr.* 2003;133(11):3428–3433.

27. Walden CE, Retzlaff BM, Buck BL, McCann BS, Knopp RH. Lipoprotein lipid response to the National Cholesterol Education Program Step II Diet by hypercholesterolemic and combined hyperlipidemic women and men. *Arterioscler Thromb Vasc Biol.* 1997; 17(2):375–382.

28. Lichtenstein AH, Asuman LM, Jalbert SM, et al. Efficacy of a Therapeutic Lifestyle Change/Step 2 diet in moderately hypercho-lesterolemic middle-aged and elderly female and male subjects. *J Lipid Res.* 2002;43(2):264–273.

29. Weitz D, Weintraub H, Fisher E, Schwartzbard AZ. Fish oil for the treatment of cardiovascular disease. *Cardiol Rev.* 2010;18(5):258–263.

30. Hu FB, Bronner L, Willett WC, et al. Fish and omega-3 fatty acid intake and risk of coronary heart disease in women. *JAMA.* 2002;287(14):1815–1821.

31. Simopoulos AP. The importance of the ratio of omega-6/omega-3 essential fatty acids. *Biomed Pharmacother.* 2002;56(8):365–379.

32. GISSI-Prevenzione Investigators (Gruppo Italiano per lo Studio della Sopravvivenza nell' Infarto miocardico). Dietary supplemen-tation with n-3 polyunsaturated fatty acids and vitamin E after myocardial infarction: results of the GISSI-Prevenzione trial. *Lancet.* 1999;354(9177):447–455.

33. Smith J. *Statin nation II: what really causes heart disease* [DVD]. 2015.

34. Messori A, Fadda V, Maratea D, Trippoli S. ω-3 fatty acid supple-ments for secondary prevention of cardiovascular disease: from "no proof of effectiveness" to "proof of no effectiveness". *JAMA Intern Med.* 2013;173(15):1466–1468. doi:10.1001/jamainternmed.2013.6638

35. Dauchet L, Amouyel P, Hercberg S, Dallongeville J. Fruit and vegeta-ble consumption and risk of coronary heart disease: a meta-analysis of cohort studies. *J Nutr.* 2006;136(10):2588–2593.

36. British Heart Foundation. *European cardiovascular disease statistics 2008.* London: British Heart Foundation; 2008.

37. Zhang X, Shu XO, Xiang YB, et al. Cruciferous vegetable consumption is associated with a reduced risk of total and cardiovascular disease mortality. *Am J Clin Nutr.* 2011;94(1):240–246. doi:10.3945/ajcn.110.009340

38. Campbell-McBride, N. *Gut and psychology syndrome.* Cambridge, U.K.: Mediform Publishing; 2004.

39. Boushey CJ, Beresford SA, Omenn GS, Motulsky AG. A quantitative assessment of plasma homocysteine as a risk factor for vascular disease. Probable benefits of increasing folic acid intakes. *JAMA.* 1995;274(13):1049–1057.

40. Bønaa K, Njølstad I, Ueland PM, et al. Homocysteine lowering and cardiovascular events after acute myocardial infarction. *N Engl J Med.* 2006;354(15):1578–1588.

41. Lonn E, Yusuf S, Arnold MJ, et al. Homocysteine lowering with folic acid and B vitamins in vascular disease. *N Engl J Med.* 2006;354(15):1567–1577.

42. Albert CM, Cook NR, Gaziano JM, et al. Effect of folic acid and B vitamins on risk of cardiovascular events and total mortality among women at high risk for cardiovascular disease: a randomized trial. *JAMA.* 2008;299(17):2027–2036.

43. Schulman SP, Becker LC, Kass DA, et al. L-Arginine therapy in acute myocardial infarction. The Vascular Interaction With Age in Myocardial Infarction (VINTAGE MI) randomized clinical trial. *JAMA.* 2006;295(1):58–64. doi:10.1001/jama.295.1.58

44. Stone I. On the genetic etiology of scurvy. *Acta Geneticae Medicae et Gemellologiae.* 1966;15:345–350.

45. Hirsch A. *Handbook of geographical and historical pathology.* Vol. II. London: The New Sydenham Society; 1885.

46. Bourne GH. Records in the older literature of tissue changes in scurvy. *Proc Royal Soc Med.* 1944;37:512–516.

47. Ebbell B. *Alt aegyptische bezeichnungen für krankheiten und symptoms.* Oslo; 1938.

48. Tröhler U. James Lind and scurvy: 1747 to 1795. JLL Bulletin: Commentaries on the history of treatment evaluation. 2013. http://www.jameslindlibrary.org/articles/james-lind-and-scurvy-1747-to-1795. Accessed March 15, 2017.

49. Cure for scurvy discovered 40 years earlier than previously thought. *Telegraph*. March 5, 2009.

50. Lodish H, Berk A, Zipursky SL, Matsudaira P, Baltimore D, Darnell JE. *Molecular cell biology, 4th edition*. New York: W.H. Freeman; 2000.

51. Alberts B, Johnson A, Lewis J, Raff R, Roberts K, Walter P. *Molecular biology of the cell, 4th edition*. New York: Garland Science; 2002.

52. Whelan MC, Senger DR. Collagen I initiates endothelial cell morphogenesis by inducing actin polymerization through suppression of cyclic AMP and protein kinase A. *J Biol Chem*. 2002;278(1):327–334. doi:10.1074/jbc.M207554200

53. Rimland B. In memoriam: Irwin Stone 1907–1984. *Journal of Orthomolecular Psychiatry*. 1984;13(4):285.

54. Stone I. *The healing factor: vitamin C against disease*. New York: Grosset and Dunlap; 1972.

55. Institute of Medicine. Food and Nutrition Board. *Dietary reference intakes for vitamin C, vitamin E, selenium, and carotenoids*. Washington, DC: National Academy Press; 2000.

56. National Institutes of Health. Vitamin C fact sheet for health professionals. https://ods.od.nih.gov/factsheets/VitaminC-Health Professional. Accessed March 15, 2017.

57. NHS Choices. Vitamin C. http://www.nhs.uk/Conditions/vitamins-minerals/Pages/Vitamin-C.aspx. Accessed March 15, 2017.

58. Tsimikas S, Hall JL. Lipoprotein(a) as a potential causal genetic risk factor of cardiovascular disease: a rationale for increased efforts to understand its pathophysiology and develop targeted therapies. *J Am Coll Cardiol*. 2012;60(8):716–721. doi:10.1016/j.jacc.2012.04.038.

59. Rath M, Pauling L. Immunological evidence for the accumulation of lipoprotein(a) in the atherosclerotic lesion of the hypoascorbemic guinea pig. *Proc Natl Acad of Sci U S A*. 1990;87(23):9388–9390.

60. Rath M, Pauling L. A unified theory of human cardiovascular disease leading the way to the abolition of this disease as a cause for human mortality. *J Ortholomol Med*. 1992;7(1):5–15.

61. Linus Pauling's Therapy®. http://www.paulingtherapy.com. Accessed March 15, 2017.

62. Knekt P, Ritz J, Pereira MA, et al. Antioxidant vitamins and coronary heart disease risk: a pooled analysis of 9 cohorts. *Am J Clin Nutr.* 2004;80(6):1508–1520.

63. Afkhami-Ardekani M, Shojaoddiny-Ardekani A. Effect of vitamin C on blood glucose, serum lipids & serum insulin in type 2 diabetes patients. *Indian J Med Res.* 2007;126(5):471–474.

64. Williams R. *Biochemical individuality.* New York: McGraw-Hill Education; 1998.

65. Elin RJ. Magnesium: the fifth but forgotten electrolyte. *Am J Clin Pathol.* 1994;102(5):616–622.

66. Takaya J, Higashino H, Kobayashi Y. Intracellular magnesium and insulin resistance. *Magnes Res.* 2004;17(2):126–136.

67. Volpe SL. Magnesium in disease prevention and overall health. *Adv Nutr.* 2013;4(3):378S–383S.

68. Dean C. *The magnesium miracle.* New York: Ballantine Books; 2006.

69. Ko YH, Hong S, Pedersen PL. Chemical mechanism of ATP synthase. Magnesium plays a pivotal role in formation of the transition state where ATP is synthesized from ADP and inorganic phosphate. *J Biol Chem.* 1999;274(41):28853–28856.

70. Douban S. Significance of magnesium in congestive heart failure. *Am Heart J.* 1996;132(3):664–671.

71. Iseri LT, French JH. Magnesium: nature's physiologic calcium blocker. *Am Heart J.* 1984;108(1):188–193.

72. Aikawa JK. *Magnesium: its biological significance.* Boca Raton, FL: CRC Press; 1981.

73. British Hypertension Society. Calcium channel blockers (CCBs) factsheet. http://www.bhsoc.org/pdfs/therapeutics/Calcium %20Channel%20Blockers%20(CCBs).pdf. Accessed March 15, 2017.

74. Jiang H, Stephens NL. Calcium and smooth muscle contraction. *Mol Cell Biochem.* 1994;135(1):1–9.

75. Lazard EM. A preliminary report on the intravenous use of magnesium sulfate in puerperal eclampsia. *Am J Obstet Gynecol.* 1925;9(4):178–188.

76. Ascherio A, Hennekens C, Willett WC, et al. Prospective study of nutritional factors, blood pressure, and hypertension among US women. *Hypertension.* 1996;27(5):1065–1072.

77. Ascherio A, Rimm EB, Giovannucci EL, et al. A prospective study of nutritional factors and hypertension among US men. *Circulation.* 1992;86(5):1475–1484.

78. Resnick LM. Oral magnesium and hypertension: research and clinical application. The Magnesium Report: Clinical, Research, and Laboratory News for Cardiologists, First Quarter 1999. http://www.mgwater.com/hyper.shtml. Accessed March 15, 2017.

79. Euser AG, Cipolla MJ. Magnesium sulfate for the treatment of eclampsia. *Stroke.* 2009;40(4):1169–1175.

80. Shechter M, Sharir M, Labrador MJ, Forrester J, Silver B, Bairey Merz CN. Oral magnesium therapy improves endothelial function in patients with coronary artery disease. *Circulation.* 2000;102(19):2353–2358.

81. National Heart Lung and Blood Institute. What is an arrhythmia? http://www.nhlbi.nih.gov/health/health-topics/topics/arr. Accessed March 15, 2017.

82. Stühlinger HG, Kiss K, Smetana R. Significance of magnesium in cardiac arrhythmias. *Wien Med Wochenschr.* 2000;150(15-16):330–334.

83. Zehender M, Meinertz T, Faber T, et al. Antiarrhythmic effects of increasing the daily intake of magnesium and potassium in patients with frequent ventricular arrhythmias. *J Am Coll Cardiol.* 1997; 29(5):1028–1034.

84. Dean C. An atrial fibrillation epidemic (blog post). http://drcarolyndean.com/2015/04/an-atrial-fibrillation-epidemic. Accessed March 15, 2017.

85. Guerrero-Romero F, Rodríguez-Morán M. Low serum magnesium levels and metabolic syndrome. *Acta Diabetol.* 2002;39(4):209–213.

86. Lopez-Ridaura R, Willett WC, Rimm EB, et al. Magnesium intake and risk of type 2 diabetes in men and women. *Diabetes Care.* 2004 Jan;27(1):134–140.

87. Seelig MS, Heggtveit HA. Magnesium interrelationships in ischemic heart disease: a review. *Am J Clin Nutr.* 1974;27(1):59–79.

88. Huges A, Tonks RS. Platelets, magnesium and myocardial infarction. *Lancet.* 1965;1(7394):1044–1046.

89. Holtmeier HJ. Magnesiumsoffwechselsstoy und Herzintarkt. In: Heilmeyer L, Holtmeier HJ, eds. *Herzinfarkt und Schoch.* Stuttgart: George Theim Verlag; 1969:110.

90. Iseri LT, Alexander LC, McCaughey RS, Boyle AJ, Myers GB. Water and electrolyte content of cardiac and skeletal muscle in heart failure and myocardial infarction. *Am Heart J.* 1952;41(2):215–227.

91. Raab W. Myocardial electrolyte derangement: crucial feature of pluricausal, so-called coronary, heart disease (dysionic cardiopathy). *Ann N Y Acad Sci.* 1969;147(17):627–686.

92. Huntsman RG, Hum BA, Lehmann H. Observations on the effect of magnesium on blood coagulation. *J Clin Pathol.* 1960;13(2):99–101.

93. Booth JV, Phillips-Bute B, McCants CB, et al. Low serum magnesium level predicts major adverse cardiac events after coronary artery bypass graft surgery. *Am Heart J.* 2003;145(6):1108–1113.

94. Rosanoff A, Weaver CM, Rude RK. Suboptimal magnesium status in the United States: are the health consequences underestimated? *Nutr Rev.* 2012;70(3):153–164.

95. Thomas D. The mineral depletion of foods available to us as a nation (1940-2002)—a review of the 6th edition of McCance and Widdowson. *Nutr Health.* 2007;19(1-2):21–55.

96. Myhill S. Magnesium: treating a deficiency. http://drmyhill.co.uk/wiki/Magnesium_-_treating_a_deficiency. Accessed March 15, 2017.

97. Browne SE. Magnesium and cardiovascular disease. *Br Med J.* 1963;2(5349):118.

98. Browne SE. The case for intravenous magnesium treatment of arterial disease in general practice: review of 34 years of experience. *J Nutr Med.* 1994;4(2)169–177.

99. Kondur AK, Hari P, Afonso LC. Complications of myocardial infarction. *Medscape.* December 18, 2014. http://emedicine.medscape.com/article/164924-overview#a3. Accessed March15, 2017.

100. Woods KL, Fletcher S, Roffe C, Haider Y. Intravenous magnesium sulphate in suspected acute myocardial infarction: results of the

second Leicester Intravenous Magnesium Intervention Trial (LIMIT-2). *Lancet*. 1992;339(8809):1553–1558.

101. Teo KK, Yusuf S, Collins R, Held PH, Peto R. Effects of intravenous magnesium in suspected acute myocardial infarction: overview of randomised trials. *BMJ*. 1991;303(6816):1499–1503.

102. Shechter M, Hod H, Marks N, Behar S, Kaplinsky E, Rabinowitz B. Beneficial effect of magnesium sulfate in acute myocardial infarction. *Am J Cardiol*. 1990;66(3):271–274.

103. Smith LF, Heagerty AM, Bing RF, Barnett DB. Intravenous infusion of magnesium sulphate after acute myocardial infarction: effects on arrhythmias and mortality. *Int J Cardiol*. 1986;12(2):175–180.

104. ISIS-4 Collaborative Group. ISIS-4: a randomized factorial trial assessing early oral captopril, oral mononitrate, and intravenous magnesium sulphate in 58,050 patients with suspected acute myocardial infarction. *Lancet*. 1995;345(8951):669–685.

105. Downing D. Is ISIS-4 research misconduct? *J Nutr Environ Med*. 1999;9:5–13.

106. World Health Organization. WHO issues new guidance on dietary salt and potassium. http://www.who.int/mediacentre/news/notes/2013/salt_potassium_20130131/en/. Accessed March 15, 2017.

107. American Heart Association. Shaking the salt habit to lower high blood pressure. http://www.heart.org/HEARTORG/Conditions/HighBloodPressure/PreventionTreatmentofHighBloodPressure/Shaking-the-Salt-Habit_UCM_303241_Article.jsp#.WMl31RAnv8M. Accessed March 15, 2017.

108. O'Donnell MJ, Mente A, Smyth A, Yusuf S. Salt intake and cardiovascular disease: why are the data inconsistent? *Eur Heart J*. 2013;34(14):1034–1040.

109. Kawasaki T, Itoh K, Uezono K, Sasaki H. A simple method for estimating 24 h urinary sodium and potassium excretion from second morning voiding urine specimen in adults. *Clin Exp Pharmacol Physiol*. 1993;20(1):7–14.

110. Smyth A, O'Donnell M, Mente A, Yusuf S. Dietary sodium and cardiovascular disease. *Curr Hypertens Rep*. 2015;17(6):559.

111. Stolarz-Skrzypek K, Kuznetsova T, Thijs L, et al. Fatal and nonfatal outcomes, incidence of hypertension, and blood pressure changes in relation to urinary sodium excretion. *JAMA*. 2011;305(17):1777–1785.

112. He FJ, MacGregor GA. Effect of modest salt reduction on blood pressure: a meta-analysis of randomized trials. Implications for public health. *J Hum Hypertens*. 2002;16(11):761–770.

113. Frost CD, Law MR, Wald NJ. By how much does dietary salt reduction lower blood pressure? II-Analysis of observational data within populations. *BMJ*. 1991;302(6780):815–818.

114. Intersalt: an international study of electrolyte excretion and blood pressure. Results for 24h urinary sodium and potassium excretion. Intersalt Cooperative Research Group. *BMJ*. 1988;297(6644):319–328.

115. Thomas MC, Moran J, Forsblom C, et al. The association between dietary sodium intake, ESRD, and all-cause mortality in patients with type 1 diabetes. *Diabetes Care*. 2011;34(4):861–866.

116. He FJ, MacGregor GA. Effect of longer-term modest salt reduction on blood pressure. *Cochrane Database Syst Rev*. 2004;(3):CD004937.

117. Cook NR, Cohen J, Hebert PR, Taylor JO, Hennekens CH. Implications of small reductions in diastolic blood pressure for primary prevention. *Arch Intern Med*. 1995;155(7):701–709.

118. Tuomilehto J, Jousilahti P, Rastenyte D, et al. Urinary sodium excretion and cardiovascular mortality in Finland. *Lancet*. 2001;357(9259):848–851.

119. Nagata C, Takatsuka N, Shimizu N, Shimizu H. Sodium intake and risk of death from stroke in Japanese men and women. *Stroke*. 2004;35(7):1543–1547.

120. Umesawa M, Iso H, Date C, Yamamoto A, et al. Relations between dietary sodium and potassium intakes and mortality from cardiovascular disease: the Japan Collaborative Cohort Study for Evaluation of Cancer Risks. *Am J Clin Nutr*. 2008;88(1):195–202.

121. He J, Ogden LG, Vupputuri S, Bazzano LA, Loria C, Whelton CK. Dietary sodium intake and subsequent risk of cardiovascular disease in overweight adults. *JAMA*. 1999;282(21):2027–2034.

122. Kagan A, Popper JS, Rhoads GG, Yano K. Dietary and other risk factors for stroke in Hawaiian Japanese men. *Stroke*. 1985;16(3):390–396.

123. Geleijnse JM, Witteman JC, Stijnen T, Kloos MW, Hofman A, Grob-bee DE. Sodium and potassium intake and risk of cardiovascular events and all-cause mortality. *Eur J Epidemiol*. 2007;22(11):763–770.

124. Tunstall-Pedoe H, Woodward M, Tavendale R, A'Brook R, McCluskey MK. Comparison of the prediction by 27 different factors of coronary heart disease and death in men and women of the Scottish Heart Health Study. *BMJ*. 1997;315(7110):722–729.

125. Yang Q, Liu T, Kuklina EV, et al. Sodium and potassium intake and mortality among US adults. *Arch Intern Med*. 2011;171(13):1183–1191.

126. Parrinello G, Di Pasquale P, Licata G, et al. Long-term effects of dietary sodium intake on cytokines and neurohormonal activation in patients with recently compensated congestive heart failure. *J Card Fail*. 2009;15(10):864–873.

127. Goyal A, Spertus JA, Gosch K, et al. Serum potassium levels and mortality in acute myocardial infarction. *JAMA*. 2012;307(2):157–164.

128. Cook NR, Obarzanek E, Cutler JA, et al. Joint effects of sodium and potassium intake on subsequent cardiovascular disease: the Trials of Hypertension Prevention follow-up study. *Arch Intern Med*. 2009;169(1):32–40.

129. Pallares DS, Rosch PJ. Magneto-metabolic therapy for advanced malignancy and cardiomyopathy. In: Rosch PJ, ed. *Bioelectromagnetic and subtle energy medicine, 2nd edition*. Boca Raton, FL: CRC Press; 2015.

130. Prasad K, Callaghan JC. Electrophysiologic basis of use of a polarizing solution in the treatment of myocardial infarction. *Clin Pharmacol Ther*. 1971;12(4):666–675.

131. Thys JP, Cornil A, Smets P, et al. Significance of the "polarizing" treatment of myocardial infarction. *Acta Cardiol*. 1974;29(1):19–29.

132. Zukowski SJ. Polarizing solutions in treatment of arrhythmias. *J Am Osteopath Assoc*. 1973;73(2):131–138.

133. Hoekenga DE, Brainard JR, Hutson JY. Rates of glycolysis and glycogenolysis during ischemia in glucose-insulin-potassium-treated perfused hearts: A 13C, 31P nuclear magnetic resonance study. *Circ Res*. 1988;62(6):1065–1074.

134. Quinones-Galvan A, Ferrannini E. Metabolic effects of glucose-insulin infusions: Myocardium and whole body. *Curr Opin Clin Nutr Metab Care.* 2001;4(2):157–163.

135. Cottin Y, Lhuillier I, Gilson L, et al. Glucose insulin potassium infusion improves systolic function in patients with chronic ischemic cardiomyopathy. *Eur J Heart Fail.* 2002;4(2):181–184.

136. Alegría Ezquerra E, Maceria González A. Therapy with glucose-insulin-potassium reduces the complications in the acute phase of myocardial infarct. Arguments in favor. *Rev Esp Cardiol.* 1998;1(9):720–726.

137. Apstein CS, Taegtmeyer H. Glucose-insulin-potassium in acute myocardial infarction: the time has come for a large, prospective trial. *Circulation.* 1997;96(4):1074–1077.

138. Apstein CS. Glucose-insulin-potassium for acute myocardial infarction: remarkable results form a new prospective, randomized trial. *Circulation.* 1998;98(21):2223–2226.

139. Díaz R, Paolasso EA, Piegas S, et al. Metabolic modulation of acute myocardial infarction. *Circulation.* 1998;98(21):2227–2234.

140. Opie LH. Proof that glucose-insulin-potassium provides metabolic protection of ischemic myocardium? *Lancet.* 1999;353(9155):768–769.

141. Khoury VK, Haluska B, Prins J, Marwick TH. Effects of glucose–insulin–potassium infusion on chronic ischaemic left ventricular dysfunction. *Heart.* 2003;89(1):61–65.

142. Sifferlin A. 90% of Americans eat too much salt. *Time Health.* Jul 02, 2015. http://time.com/3944545/sodium-heart/. Accessed March 15, 2017.

143. Sabaroff R. Home soil, season 1, episode 18 (television episode). *Star Trek: The Next Generation.* Los Angeles: Paramount Television; 1988.

144. Chan J, Knutsen SF, Blix GG, Lee JW, Fraser GE. Water, other fluids, and fatal coronary heart disease: the Adventist Health Study. *Am J Epidemiol.* 2002;155(9):827–833.

145. Becker RC. The role of blood viscosity in the development and progression of coronary artery disease. *Cleve Clin J Med.* 1993;60(5):353–358.

146. Lowe GD, Lee AJ, Rumley A, Price JF, Fowkes FG. Blood viscosity and risk of cardiovascular events: the Edinburgh Artery Study. *Br J Haematol.* 1997;96(1):168–173.

147. Lee AJ, Mowbray PI, Lowe GD, Rumley A, Fowkes FG, Allan PL. Blood viscosity and elevated carotid intima-media thickness in men and women. *Circulation*. 1998;97(15):1467–1473.

148. Koenig W, Ernst E. The possible role of hemorheology in athero-thrombogenesis. *Atherosclerosis*. 1992;94(2 3):93 107.

149. Becker RC. Seminars in thrombosis, thrombolysis, and vascular biology. Part 5. Cellular-rheology and plasma viscosity. *Biorheology*. 1991;79(4):265–270.

150. Ernst E. Hematocrit and cardiovascular risk. *J Intern Med*. 1995;237 (6):527–528.

151. de Simone G, Devereux RB, Chien S, Alderman MH, Atlas SA, Laragh JH. Relation of blood viscosity to demographic and physiologic variables and to cardiovascular risk factors in apparently normal adults. *Circulation*. 1990;81(1):107–117.

152. Erikssen G, Thaulow E, Sandvik L, Stormorken H, Erikssen J. Haematocrit: a predictor of cardiovascular mortality? *J Intern Med*. 1993;234(5):493–499.

153. Lowe GD, Drummond MM, Lorimer AR, et al. Relation between extent of coronary artery disease and blood viscosity. *Br Med J*. 1980;280(6215):673–674.

154. Ciuffetti G, Schillaci G, Lombardini R, Pirro M, Vaudo G, Mannarino E. Prognostic impact of low-shear whole blood viscosity in hypertensive men. *Eur J Clin Invest*. 2005;35(2):93–98.

155. Seaman GV, Engel R, Swank RL, Hissen W. Circadian periodicity in some physicochemical parameters of circulating blood. *Nature*. 1965;207(999):833–835.

156. Okamura K, Washimi Y, Endo H, et al. Can high fluid intake prevent cerebral and myocardial infarction? Systematic review. *Nihon Ronen Igakkai Zasshi*. 2005;42(5):557–563.

157. Warren JL, Bacon WE, Harris T, McBean AM, Foley DJ, Phillips C. Burden and outcomes associated with dehydration among US elderly, 1991. *Am J Public Health*.1994;84(8):1265–1269.

158. Cohen MC, Muller JE. Onset of acute myocardial infarction—circadian variation and triggers. *Cardiovasc Res*. 1992;26(9):831–838.

159. Toiler GH, Brezinski D, Schafer AI, et al. Concurrent morning increase in platelet aggregability and the risk of myocardial infarction and sudden cardiac death. *N Engl J Med*. 1987;316(24):1514–1518.

160. Neuhäuser-Berthold M, Beine S, Verwied SC, Lührmann PM. Coffee consumption and total body water homeostasis as measured by fluid balance and bioelectrical impedance analysis. *Ann Nutr Metab*. 1997;41(1):29–36.

161. Kobayashi J. On geographical relationship between the chemical nature of river water and death-rate from apoplexy. *Bar Ohara Inst Landwirt Biol*. 1957:11;12–21.

162. Schroeder HA. Relation between mortality from cardiovascular disease and treated water supplies: variations in states and 163 largest municipalities of the United States. *J Am Med Assoc*. 1960:172;1902–1908.

163. Anderson TW, Neri LC, Schreiber GB, Talbot FD, Zdrojewski A. Letter: Ischemic heart disease, water hardness and myocardial magnesium. *Can Med Assoc J*. 1975;113(3):199–203.

164. Masironi R, Piša Z, Clayton D. Myocardial infarction and water hardness in the WHO myocardial infarction registry network. *Bull World Health Organ*. 1979;57(2):291–299.

165. Leoni V, Fabiani L, Ticchiarelli L. Water hardness and cardiovascular mortality rate in Abruzzo, Italy. *Arch Environ Health*. 1985;40(5):274–278.

166. Sengupta P, Sahoo S. A cross sectional study to evaluate the fitness pattern among the young fishermen of Coastal Orissa. *Indian J Public Health Research and Development*. 2013;4(1):171–175.

167. Kubis M. Relation of water hardness to the occurrence of acute myocardial infarct. *Acta Univ Palacki Olomuc Fac Med*. 1985;111:321–324.

168. Anderson TW, Leriche WH, Hewitt D, Neri LC. Magnesium, water hardness, and heart disease. In: Itokawa Y, Durlach J, eds. *Magnesium in health and disease*. New Barnet: John Libbey Press; 1989: 565–571.

Chapter Eight: Conclusion: What to Do

1. Taubes G. *Why we get fat*. New York: Alfred A. Knopf; 2010.

2. Harcombe Z. *The obesity epidemic: what caused it? How can we stop it?* Monmouthshire: Columbus Publishing; 2015.

3. Lustig R. *Fat chance: the hidden truth about sugar, obesity, and disease.* London: Fourth Estate; 2014.

4. Teicholz N. *The big fat surprise: why butter, meat, and cheese belong in a healthy diet.* New York: Simon & Schuster; 2015.

5. Noakes T, Proudfoot J, Creed S. *The real meal revolution: the radical, sustainable approach to healthy eating.* London: Robinson; 2015.

6. Foster GD, Wyatt HR, Hill JO, et al. A randomized trial of a low-carbohydrate diet for obesity. *N Eng J Med.* 2003;348(21):2082–2090.

7. Shai I, Schwarzfuchs D, Henkin Y, et al. Weight loss with a low-carbohydrate, Mediterranean, or low-fat diet. *N Eng J Med.* 2008;359(3):229–241.

8. Brehm BJ, Seeley RJ, Daniels SR, et al. A randomized trial comparing a very low carbohydrate diet and a calorie-restricted low fat diet on body weight and cardiovascular risk factors in healthy women. *J Clin Endocrinol Metab.* 2003;88(4):1617–1623.

9. Stern L, Iqbal N, Seshadri P, et al. The effects of low-carbohydrate versus conventional weight loss diets in severely obese adults: one-year follow-up of a randomized trial. *Ann Intern Med.* 2004;140(10):778–785.

10. Yancy WS, Olsen MK, Guyton JR, Bakst RP, Westman EC. A low-carbohydrate, ketogenic diet versus a low-fat diet to treat obesity and hyperlipidemia. *Ann Intern Med.* 2004;140(10):769–777.

11. Gardner CD, Kiazand A, Alhassan S, et al. Comparison of the Atkins, Zone, Ornish and LEARN diets for change in weight and related risk factors among overweight premenopausal women. *JAMA.* 2007;297(9):969–977.

12. Garg A, Bantle JP, Henry RR, et al. Effects of varying carbohydrate content of diet in patients with non-insulin-dependent diabetes mellitus. *JAMA.* 1994;271(18):1421–1428.

13. Samaha FF, Iqbal N, Seshadri P, et al. A low-carbohydrate as compared with a low-fat diet in severe obesity. *N Engl J Med.* 2003;348(21):2074–2081.

14. Freemantle N, Holmes J, Hockey A, Kumar S. How strong is the association between abdominal obesity and the incidence of type 2 diabetes? *Int J Clin Pract.* 2008;62(9):1391–1396.

15. National Heart, Lung, and Blood Institute. What is diabetic heart disease? https://www.nhlbi.nih.gov/health/health-topics/topics/dhd. Accessed March 15, 2017.

16. Myers J, Prakash M, Froelicher V, Do D, Partington S, Atwood JE. Exercise capacity and mortality among men referred for exercise testing. *N Engl J Med.* 2002;346(11):793–801.

17. Borghouts LB, Keizer HA. Exercise and insulin sensitivity: a review. *Int J Sports Med.* 2000;21(1):1–12.

18. Siegel AJ, Januzzi J, Sluss P, et al. Cardiac biomarkers, electrolytes, and other analytes in collapsed marathon runners: implications for the evaluation of runners following competition. *Am J Clin Pathol.* 2008;129(6):948–951.

19. British Heart Foundation. *Coronary heart disease statistics 2015.* London: British Heart Foundation; 2015.

20. Niedermaier ON, Smith ML, Beightol LA, Zukowska-Grojec Z, Goldstein DS, Eckberg DL. Influence of cigarette smoking on human autonomic function. *Circulation.* 1993;88(2):562–571.

21. Middlekauff HR, Park J, Moheimani RS. Adverse effects of cigarette and noncigarette smoke exposure on the autonomic nervous system: mechanisms and implications for cardiovascular risk. *J Am Coll Cardiol.* 2014;64(16):1740–1750.

INDEX

Page numbers in *italics* refer to photographs and figures; page numbers followed by *t* refer to tables.

ABOUT THE AUTHOR

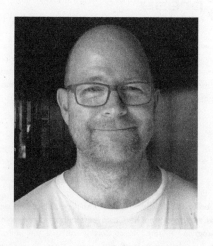

JUSTIN SMITH is the producer, director, and writer of the documentaries *Statin Nation I* and *II*. He was formerly a personal trainer, sports massage therapist, and nutrition coach. The documentaries arose from a general-nutrition book planned by Justin. He originally hoped to only spend one chapter on cholesterol but rerouted the entire project once the overwhelming evidence disillusioned his notions of heart disease. He is based in the United Kingdom.

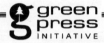

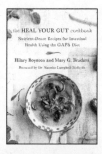
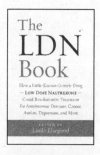
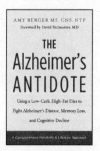
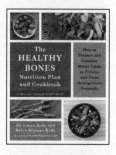
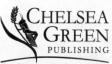

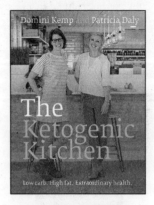
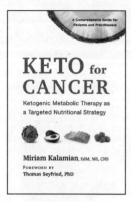
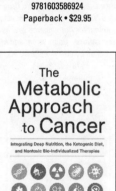
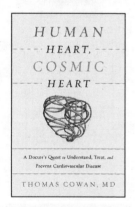
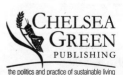